FIGHT BREAST CANCER

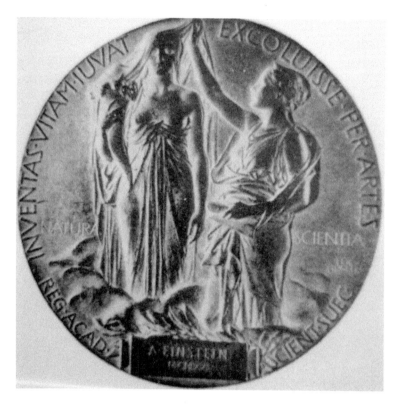

EINSTEIN NOBLE GOLD MEDAL PRIZE SHOWS
SCIENCE UNVEILS SECRETS OF NATURE

PARVIS GAMAGAMI, MD

Copyright © 2016 Parvis Gamagami
All rights reserved
First Edition

PAGE PUBLISHING, INC.
New York, NY

First originally published by Page Publishing, Inc. 2016

ISBN 978-1-68213-784-0 (pbk)
ISBN 978-1-68213-785-7 (digital)

Printed in the United States of America

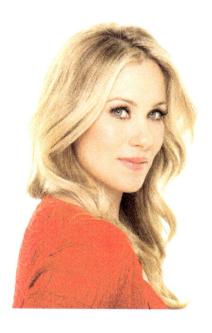

'When I was 9 years old I watched my mom hear the words "you have breast cancer" she dropped the phone. In 1995 I watched as she dealt with ovarian cancer. She is now 74. My wonderful doctor George Weinberger made sure I was tested since the age of 30. He sent me to Dr Gamagami. For years I just had mammograms. And then my sweet Parvis suggested an MRI. BECAUSE My breasts were dense. They saw something and did a biopsy. It was nothing. So three months later I had to go for a follow up and I had DCIS in the other breast. With some invasive cells. If not for dr Gamagami. I would not be alive   I am BRCA positive. And I know of my risks. This book is so informative on many levels. From food to lifestyle to genetics to underwire bras. We must be mindful.'

Christina Applegate, Sadie's mama

To my dear wife, Lili, with love

DISCLAIMER

The author of this book does not have any relation with any financial supporter, has no financial interest in any form, with any pharmaceutical product or any type of laboratories.

FIGHT NEW WAYS BREAST CANCER: A GUIDE TO FIND OUT MATERIAL DISCUSSED IN THIS BOOK

In order to efficiently fight breast cancer, our voracious and tricky enemy, we should know everything about it, when and how it attacks and when and how we should fight back.

If you want to know how and where to make the most appropriate investigation of breast cancer, look at chapter 1.

If you want to know how important is the date of the menstrual cycle in the management of breast cancer and breast physiology, look at chapter 2.

If you want to know how breast cancer is born, look at chapter 3.

If you want to know how breast cancer develops and spreads metastasis, look at chapter 4.

If you want to know about the risk of bilateral breast cancer, look at chapter 5.

If you want to know what the risk factors are of breast cancer, look at chapter 6.

If you want to know about the debatable and untold risk factor of breast cancer, look at chapter 7.

If you want to know how we detect breast cancer, look at chapter 8.

If you want to know how breast cancer is diagnosed, look at chapter 9.

If you want to know about the classic treatment of breast cancer, surgery, radiation, side effects, look at chapter 10.

If you want to know about chemotherapy, anti-hormone therapy, and risk-benefit, look at chapter 11.

If you want to know why breast cancer recurs, what it means, and how it can be prevented, look at chapter 12.

If you want to know about male breast cancer and its difference with the female breast cancer, look at chapter 13.

If you want to know if our treatment impacts the decline of mortality of breast cancer, look at chapter 14.

If you want to know how genetics revolutionized management of breast cancer, look at chapter 15.

If you want to know about harmless conservative treatments and alternatives to classic treatment of breast cancer, look at chapter 16.

If you want to know how treated breast cancer can be followed up, look at chapter 17.

If you want to know about final notes, survival of breast cancer, and if breast cancer can be prevented /or cured, look at chapter 18.

GLOSSARY

Aneuploidy: Abnormal number of chromosomes

Angiogenesis: Formation of blood vessels

Arm Lymphedema: Swelling of arm due to the obstruction of lymphatic channels

Carcinocidal: Killing cancer

Carcinogenic: Causing cancer

Clinically: Medically

Conservative Treatment of Breast Cancer: No mastectomy; preservation of breast, removal of cancer alone (lumpectomy) with or without radiation

Core Needle Biopsy: Taking wormlike sample from a lesion by special needle

DCIS: Ductal carcinoma in situ, early stage of breast cancer confined inside of milk ducts

DNA: Abbreviation for deoxyribonucleic acid, a chemical substance forming genes

Edema: Accumulation of water in tissue

Epigenic Mutation: Change of molecular expression of DNA

Erythema: Red irritation of the skin

Fibrosis: Scar formed by reaction of fibrotic tissue

Fluoroscopy: Examination of internal organs by x-rays

FNA: Fine needle aspiration, cell aspiration from a lesion by ordinary needle and syringe for microscopic examination

Gene: Chemical material carrying predetermined plans for organ formation and their function

Hematogenic: Originating from blood

Hematoma: Well-walled blood collection.

Hyperplasia: Increased benign cell proliferations

Keloid: Thick red-colored scar on the skin

LCIS: Lobular carcinoma in situ; multiplication of the cells in the lobules of milk gland, per se is not a cancer but high risk for cancer

Likenification: Post-irritation of thickened skin scar

Lumpectomy: Removal of a lump

Lymphogenic: Originating from lymphatic system

Macrocalcifications: Minute particles of calcium deposited in the tissue due to destruction of the cells

Mastectomy: Removal of the breast

Metastasis: Local or distant spread of cancer

Mutation: Molecular change in the gene

Nanotechnology: Technique using particles of one billionth of a meter

Neoangiogenesis: Formation of new vessels by cancer

Neoductogenesis: Formation of new milk ducts by cancer

Oncogene: Chemical causing cancer of the cell

Palliative Treatment: Temporary remedy, not curative treatment

Peau d'Orange: Orange peel aspect seen in inflammatory breast cancer

Peritumoral Lipogenesis: Formation of fatty tissue around the cancer

Placebo: Fictitious test or no treatment

Pneumothorax Treatment: Old treatment of lung tuberculosis by injecting air in the pleural space, collapsing the lung, healing tuberculotic cavities, performing numerous checkups by x-rays

Prophylactic Treatment: Preventive treatment

Proto-oncogene: Precancerous gene

Randomized Trial: Assigned one group to an experimental test comparing the results with a similar group without treatment or placebo

Sporadic Cancer: Cancer occurring in general population without family history of breast cancer

Stereotactic Core Needle Biopsy: Special x-ray machine which can determine the depth of the lesion for core needle biopsy

Symptom: Group of signs in a disease.

Syndrome: Group of symptoms in a disease

Telangiectasia: Formation of minute new vessels on the skin exposed to irradiation

Thrombosis: Clot formation in a vessel

Trisomia: Triplet chromosomes

OUR HIPPOCRATIC OATH: PRIMUM NON NOCERE (DO NO HARM)

The purpose of medicine:

1. Prevent disease.
2. If we cannot prevent it, cure it.
3. If we cannot cure it, prolong life without harm.

In matters of breast cancer,

Can we prevent it? If not, can we cure it?

If not, can we prolong life without harm?

Is there a better way to treat breast cancer than the present ones?

Readers will find truthful answers to those questions in this book.

Breast cancer is more frightening than dangerous despite the fact that the occurrence of breast cancer does not cause fatality at its onset; it is more fearful than heart attack and brain stroke, which carry high mortality at the onset or leave serious disabilities in its aftermath. Other cancers, before their diagnosis, manifest by pain, fatigue, fever, loss of appetite, loss of weight, bleeding, anemia, cognitive dysfunction, etc. Breast cancer lives with the patient peacefully for years without any sign before its detection. In majority of the cases, when diagnosed, it behaves like a chronic disease, with ups and downs. A patient with breast cancer is not a sick person. She becomes sick from the time that she gets undesirable news of the breast biopsy, cancer. Then she becomes quite sick from the thought of cancer, controversies of opinion of the treatment, fear of surgical complications, deformity of the breast, side effect of radiation therapy, toxicity of the chemotherapy, losing hair, all leading to a chronic distress, worse than cancer itself. The patient has to fight in two fronts: one against breast cancer, the second against the side effect of our treatment. In published books by health providers for the public, they talk mainly of cure and goodness of our treatment, but their side effects are either minimized or not mentioned. In my experience even a large number of physicians and by and large the public don't know the exact amount of side effects of our present treatments of breast cancer, which should be explained before any treatment of our patients. Today, patients participate more actively in their treatment of breast cancer than before. They are also more sophisticated. They are the offspring of the computer generation reaching the age of booming breast cancer.

They want and they must know everything in each step of their treatment and must have precise information of the result of the new research of new concepts. A young patient was told that she has a 5 cm breast cancer, stage III; she needs a mastectomy, then radiation, and after that chemotherapy. This news was devastating for her. In desperation, searching in libraries and computer aids, she found out that there was another way of assessment that can tell her that she might not need either mastectomy, radiation, nor chemotherapy and that she can preserve her breast and be treated only by simple removal of the mass from the breast. That was new information from genetic tests. For prolongation of life, some breast cancer need harsh treatment that can cause severe side effects; for some other breast cancer, that treatment is unnecessary.

If we don't provide precise information about breast cancer, how do we expect patients to make a correct, informed consent and an informed decision? In order to obtain optimum result in the management of breast cancer, first we as physicians ought to know all new scientific acquisitions and communicate them to our patients.

SUMMARY OF EIGHTEEN CHAPTERS IN THIS BOOK

The intention of writing this book is to provide and make the public aware of recent discoveries in genetics of breast cancer that revolutionized our three-thousand-year concept of natural history of breast cancer and its treatment. In order to fight our enemy, breast cancer, first of all we should know it well. Here, it is shown how and where it is born, how it spreads (malignant cells to distant organs), what the risk factors are for its birth, how we find it, how we treat it and what the results are, and why a patient with early stage cancer (stage I) with surgery, radiotherapy, chemotherapy passes away in three years and another patient with advanced breast cancer of 5 cm in size (stage III) without radiotherapy and chemotherapy lives another twenty-five years. Replacing conservative treatment (preservation of the breast, removing only breast cancer, axillary lymph node dissection, breast irradiation) with radical mastectomy (chest wall mutilation) in the last century was a big leap; this became the standard of early breast cancer treatment. However, this type of treatment is not without harms and serious side effects well documented in the literature and added more graphically by author's observations on supervising four thousand treated breast cancers.

The twenty-first century is a new era in the breast cancer management based on genetic findings of breast cancer. In this book, it is shown that now it is possible to treat breast cancer while preserving the breast, without axillary lymph node dissection and breast irradiation, eliminating side effects, through harmless alternative treatment of breast cancer with better survival and high satisfaction of patients.

THE PURPOSE OF THIS BOOK

Many books have been written about breast cancer for the public by breast cancer survivors reciting the ordeal of their breast cancer journey. Books written by surgeons and oncologists are informative but always advocating the same stereotypic classic treatment without challenging their efficacy or proposing any new approach to the treatment of breast cancer.

One interesting book was published in 1970 by Dr. George Crile *What Women Should Know about Breast Cancer Controversies*. He was vilified by his colleagues because he said mastectomy, axillary lymph node dissection, and breast radiation are unnecessary in breast cancer. Was he wrong? Or did he make a prophetic statement more than forty years ago? You will see later what today's genetic science and clinical randomization trials have shown in that subject. In this book, every statement is documented by a graphic demonstration (a picture is worth a hundred words), and you will find many untold and unknown events that occurred during my fifty-five years of practice in the field of breast cancer. I want to share my experience with the public and my colleagues. Science and technology have progressed so fast in the last decade in our field, which has created a large gap even among physicians in this field. New acquisitions still remain unknown to many practitioners. The gap is much bigger between scientific knowledge and the public perceptions. The more correct information we provide to our patients, the better we prepare them to fight breast cancer. Our mission is to inform the patients with honesty the success and the failure of our methods of diagnosis and treatment of breast cancer and submit them to the least stressful and harmful management of breast cancer and avoid unnecessary harsh procedures because the standards say so. We are members of a supportive group providing emotional and moral support to our patients and also servant companions in their ordeal of breast cancer journey. Isn't it our raison d'être?

In this book a minimum of necessary updated information published in the literature and personal experience are provided for awareness of who are interested in the matter of breast cancer. This is a platform for patients with recent diagnosis of breast cancer. With these information patients can discuss with their physicians while knowing beforehand the pros and cons of proposed treatment.

Any health provider in the field of radiology, surgery, gynecology, and internal medicine, medical residents, nursing students, and the public can obtain in a few hours all proven and documented information about modern method of diagnosis and treatment of breast cancer.

GENERAL INFORMATION

Status Quo of Cancer

Cancer is the biggest health problem of human beings. In the USA one of two men and one of three women catch cancer that should be treated for a very long time. Actually, there are 13 million cancer survivors; more than 1.5 million of them survive for more than twenty years. One of every four deaths is due to cancer (25% of deaths).

Breast cancer: At the present time, 3 million breast cancer patients survive, 2 million are treated for breast cancer, and 1 million carry breast cancer without knowing it. Each year in the USA more than two hundred thousand breast cancer is diagnosed and forty thousand females lose their lives. Is it because we diagnose breast cancer too late? Or we don't have the medication to cure it? Treatment of breast cancer is very expensive—more than $25 billion a year. Is it because of overtreatment or inadequate treatment? Worldwide, each year over 1.5 million new breast cancer cases develop. All nations in the world look at the USA as the world leader in the fight for breast cancer. At the present time, not only is the standard of detection and treatment of breast cancer hardly affordable in the USA, the richest nation in the world, but also it is impossible to be duplicated technically, medically, or financially in the rest of the world.

The public *world health organization* sees our present policy in the management of breast cancer impracticable, toxic, and extraordinarily costly that cannot help the vast majority of women in the world at risk of developing breast cancer. Do we have any answer to this problem? Today, in the twenty-first century we are able to detect breast cancer earlier, sooner, and smaller than the last century. But still the standard of treatment of early breast cancer is practiced on the same concept of the last century (one size fits all). The large number of noninvasive or invasive breast cancer with no aggressivity is overtreated because we do not know which ones were aggressive and which were nonaggressive. For a century we have been dreaming of being able to differentiate an aggressive breast cancer from a nonaggressive one. In the eve of the last century and in the beginning of the twenty-first century, by discovery of genetics in breast cancer, those dreams become true. Genetic findings revolutionized the concept of natural history of breast cancer and established a new set of mind and new standards in the treatment of breast cancer. Now we know which cancer is low-aggressive, and this is a real breakthrough, avoiding overtreatment, which is so expensive for the patients and for the society.

The author reports in this book his long experience with breast cancer and describes all side effects and harms of our present treatment published in the literature, which led him to formulate an alternative harmless treatment of breast cancer based on genetic findings with much better life quality and same survival benefit but less cost for society.

CONTRIBUTION OF AMERICAN WOMEN TO THE NOBLE CAUSE

American women deserve international praise. American women were and are pioneers in the war against breast cancer. They deserve the biggest worldwide credit and recognition. American women have saved the lives of millions of females in the world with relentless effort lobbying in the congress for passing legislation for screening mammography; otherwise, we would not have been followed by other nations and be saving millions of female lives worldwide. Screening mammography legislation not only showed its efficiency in detection of early breast cancer and consequently curbing mortality but also opened the door to the greatest medical industries, creating thousands of jobs around the world. Medical engineering led to the discovery of digital mammography, breast MRI, high-tech ultrasonography, breast nuclear medicine for diagnosis and treatment, a large variety of surgical procedures, reconstruction, mammoplasty, silicone, saline bag industry, industry of radiation therapy high kilo voltage, brachytherapy, intraoperative target therapy, and lastly, genetic industry in breast cancer. Still, American women actively continue in organizing mass manifestation for more research to find the cause of breast cancer and to wipe it out from our lives. They are supported and appreciated by the entire world. Thanks to the American women.

BIOGRAPY OF THE AUTHOR

After graduating from Sorbonne, Paris, France, in 1947, he was admitted to the Medical School of Paris University of Descartes. On the first day of his medical training he was assigned to the department of radiotherapy in Curie Institute—one of the most prestigious cancer centers in Europe. At that time, radiation therapy of the breast was a hot topic in Europe, particularly in France because in Curie Institute under the direction of his first mentor, Dr. Baclasse, for the first time in the world he tried to treat breast cancer with radiation alone, without surgery. In the first year of his medical school he was so impressed with the good result of radiation in inoperable breast cancer leftover of the surgeons that he decided to become a radiologist. At that time, diagnostic radiology and radiotherapy were together one specialty. It should be mentioned that medical education in France at that time was Napoleon-type of training, delivering wartime physicians, even specialists.

In 1954, he graduated as a medical doctor. In 1963 he received his diploma of specialty in radiology and radiotherapy and, in 1972, a professorship assignment in radiology. He was fortunate to have many years of fellowship in radiology and radiotherapy in Sweden, nuclear medicine in England, and breast disease in France in Strasbourg. His medical residency in the USA, fellowship in Europe, and experience in both worlds enhanced his vision and taught him how to use the best of each medicine in the care of his patients in the last thirty years in the USA. His fifty-five years of medical practice in the matter of breast cancer is divided in two parts. Twenty-five years were spent abroad in academic positions at different universities as a professor of radiology, practicing and teaching diagnostic and radiotherapy of the breast, and the last thirty years practicing in the USA in specialized comprehensive breast center in Van Nuys and in the breast care center in Encino (RadNet), California.

In 1963 in France, breast cancer was recognized as a specialty. A specialist was called a senologist (*senos* in Latin means "breast")—a breast physician/doctor being in contact with the patient, in fact a primary care breast physician (clinician radiologist). These physicians were trained and certified in diagnostic radiology and radiotherapy, trained on how to perform a physical examination, interpret mammography and other imaging techniques, perform ultrasonography, perform fine needle aspiration of the breast for diagnosis and treatment, interpret aspirated cytology slides, perform superficial biopsy and punch biopsy, treat a cyst, abscess, and breast infection, do radiotherapy of the breast cancer, and conduct breast consultation and follow up patients after treatment. This type of practice provided the highest level of satisfaction and was the most economical for patients and society and scientific progression in the breast diseases.

His practice and personal experience in the last thirty years in comprehensive breast centers Because of his background in breast oncology, contact with a thousand patients, physical examination, and consultation were an integral part of his daily practice. He continued his practice the same way.

His experience consists of the following:

1. Taking care of 170,000 patients, personally examining clinically each of them, correlating physical examination with their imaging findings of the breast; this is one of the largest number of patients having a complete breast examination by a single physician.
2. Interpreting mammography, over 650,000.
3. Performing stereotactic core needle biopsy, over 3,500.

4. Performing fine needle biopsy for diagnosis and treatment of cysts, over 21,000.

5. Performing ultrasonography, over 40,000.

6. Performing ductography, over 1,000.

7. Clinical radiological follow up of 4,000 breast cancer, from two years to up to thirty years.

8. Consultation, review of mammography, MRI, second opinion for diagnosis, and treatment of breast cancer, over 3,500.

Scientific contribution of the author to the medical literature reported for the first time and published in his book *Atlas of Mammography* (1996) and in the present book:

1. Mammographic demonstration of angiogenesis and identification of proper nutrient artery of breast cancer; important for detection of earliest stage of breast cancer.

2. Mammographic demonstration of sequences of evolution of undefined precancerous image to defined image of cancer; important for detection of early stage of breast cancer.

3. Mammographic demonstration of peritumoral lipogenesis of breast cancer; this cancer mimics breast lipoma. It is important for physicians to be aware of such entity and not to be misled.

4. Demonstration of neoductogenesis of intraductal carcinoma in situ (DCIS) by ductography; important for determination of extension of DCIS.

5. Endoductal neoangiogenesis discovered by immunostaining technique in DCIS; very important in predicting the risk of metastasis in DCIS.

6. Progressive breast retraction of the breast cancer treated with irradiation due to recurrent cancer mimicking post-radiation fibrosis; it is important for physicians not to be mistaken.

7. Stereotactic core needle biopsy targeting lesion combined with ductography.

8. Bracketing hooked wires technique; for total excision of breast cancer with large clear margins should be obtained at first surgical attempt.

9. Ductectomy; resection of sick ducts by ductography with multiple hook wire localization.

10. Documentation of breast trauma and breast cancer.

11. Documentation of untold damages of underwire brassiere and breast cancer relation.

12. Documentation of side effects of breast irradiation twenty-five years after treatment.

13. Presentation of harmless treatment of breast cancer based on genetic findings.

How were they practicing in olden days?

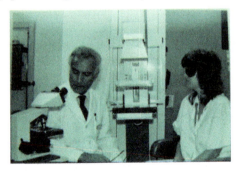

It is good to know how clinician radiologists or breast care physicians called senologists were practicing and taking care of breast disease fifty years ago in the old continent in the offices or hospital-based clinics.

Self- or physician-referred patients were examined by necessary diagnostic means such as physical examination, mammography, ultrasonography, galactography, and fine needle breast exploration, reading slides of aspirated cells of the lesion. At the end of the session the patient was informed of the results of the tests and plan of the treatment, and follow-ups were proposed and discussed.

For example, a patient found a painful nodule in her breast.

First, patient underwent physical examination, then diagnostic procedures.

If painful nodule proved to be a cyst by ultrasonography and totally collapsed after fine needle aspiration of the fluid, patient would be discharged—no further treatment.

If painful nodule proved to be an abscess by ultrasonography and pussy material found by fine needle aspiration and cytology inflammatory cells in instantaneous slide reading, antibiotics would be prescribed—no further treatment. Large abscess would have been referred to a surgeon.

If painful nodule proved to be a solid mass by ultrasonography and on mammography an undetermined mass density, if fine needle aspiration cytology showed typical for adenoma or atypia for malignancy, patient would be referred to a surgeon. Patient would be followed up after treatment of breast cancer.

This shortcut, saving time and abating anxiety, which is immensely satisfactory for the patient, is extremely economical for society and highly efficient in the care of breast discomfort when compared with present norms of breast care.

Even today, according to the author, that type of care for breast disease is needed more than ever before.

CHAPTER 1

WHERE AND WHO MAKE APPROPRIATE INVESTIGATION OF BREAST CANCER

BIRTH OF NEW SPECIALTY

In olden days, a physician could practice all branches of medicine encompassing surgery, internal medicine, obstetrics, pediatrics, ophthalmology, etc. Our license still has the titles physician and Surgeon.

In less than half a century, more than one hundred medical specialties and subspecialties have been born. In fact, medicine is directed toward organ specialties and subspecialties. One of them is the breast cancer specialty. Breast cancer specialty has emerged because of the necessity and advancement in medicine. As a matter of fact, breast cancer is such a vast disease that dominates all other diseases of the breast. Today, detection of breast cancer and its treatment requires teamwork under one roof of many specialists (called Comprehensive Breast Center).

FIRST COMPREHENSIVE BREAST CENTER IN THE WORLD

Charles Gros (1910-1984)

The first comprehensive breast center was created in 1963 in Strasbourg (France) by Charles Gros, professor of mathematics, physician, radiologist, radiotherapist, and inventor of French molybdenum target senograph machine in use all over the world for mammography. He founded a unique comprehensive breast center composed of the department of radiodiagnostic mammography, ultrasonography, department of pathology, and department of radiotherapy, nuclear medicine, psychology, and plastic surgery all under one roof in the heart of a 3,000-bed city hospital staffed by physicians of the University of Pasteur of Strasburg.

His center became a medical mecca for breast cancer care. Thousands of radiologists and surgeons from all over the world flocked to this center to be taught methodology of breast cancer diagnosis and mainly conservative treatment, lumpectomy, and radiation, which was very much advocated at that time in France. Thousands of breast cancer patients from many countries were referred to this center for treatment. Charles Gros was a man ahead of his time with unusual wisdom. His motto in breast cancer was to treat the mind before the body. His clinical view, advice for breast cancer detection, and technique of conservative treatment and follow-up, for more than half a century, have not been outdated as of today. I should mention that in France, sooner than any other nation, breast disease was recognized as a medical specialty called senology. Also, a society of senologists was founded by Charles Gros in 1963. Later, relatively similar societies were created, such as the Society of Mastology in South America and Breast Imaging Society in the USA, and because of the importance and the vast pathology of breast disease and breast cancer and advancement in technology in the last decade, a fellowship in breast imaging has been organized by some medical schools in the USA which has played a great role in detection of breast cancer and curbing the mortality.

FIRST COMPREHENSIVE BREAST CENTER IN THE USA, CONCEPT OF A TEAMWORK—VAN NUYS, CALIFORNIA

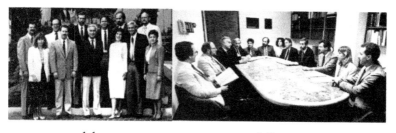

1.1 1.2

Medical staff, 12 breast specialists   Weekly tumor board of medical staff

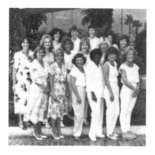

1.3

Nursing and technologist staff

The first comprehensive center in the USA, a free-standing multidisciplinary institution, was founded in 1982 by Dr. Melvin Silverstein, a man of great vision heading a team composed of seven specialists with a background of five to twenty-five years of experience in the matter of breast cancer. Surgical oncologist, medical oncologist, plastic surgeon, clinician radiologist, radiotherapist, pathologist, and psychologist equipped with surgical suite, operating room, radiology department, pathology suite, and over thirty staff personnel. In our first five years we had more than one hundred visitors from all over the world to see the new concept of comprehensive breast center and management of breast cancer, particularly conservative treatment for breast cancer with or without radiotherapy. And à propos of patients: once patients came to our breast center and had great satisfaction, they continued to return year after year from many states, either for routine checkup or continued follow-up. The number of patients increased regularly. Seven to nine thousand patients booked their appointments a year ahead for their next visit. The large majority of our patients were self-referred by word of mouth.

Self- or physician-referred patients if symptomatic were seen first by the surgeon. Otherwise, all patients were seen by the clinician radiologist (author). After physical examination, the patient had a mammography, then, if necessary, ultrasonography, fine needle aspiration, or core needle biopsy—all performed often in one session. The result was communicated to the patient before leaving the premises. If the patient had any questions, they were answered. If she wanted to see her mammography, it was shown to her and explained in detail by the radiologist. All type of diagnostic procedures, imaging, localization biopsy, surgery, pathology, chemotherapy, and consultation with the radiotherapist or psychologist were performed in our center under one roof. There was no need for the patient to go elsewhere. If the patient needed special treatment, her file would be discussed in our weekly tumor board in the presence of all specialists. Treatment would be planned and performed the following days in our facility.

One of the most succinct textbooks about breast cancer was published in France by Charles Gros ten years after the inauguration of this comprehensive breast center in Strasburg. In our case, after a relatively short period of time, we discovered more early stages of noninvasive breast cancer DCIS (394 cases) than any institution in the world, thus contributing to our much better knowledge of natural history of breast cancer and early mammographic breast cancer detection, which formed the basis of a textbook published fourteen years later titled *Atlas of Mammography: New Early Sign of Breast Cancer* by Parvis Gamagami, MD, in 1996. The result obtained in the treatment of DCIS with and without radiation therapy in our center formed the basis of another textbook published sixteen years later by Mel Silverstein, MD, called *Ductal Carcinoma In Situ* in 1998, a unique book among its kind and entirely dedicated to DCIS with participation of international experts. At the same time, more than fifty articles about breast cancer were also published in prestigious medical journals.

HOW BREAST CANCER IS DETECTED AND TREATED OUTSIDE OF COMPREHENSIVE BREAST CENTERS, WHICH IS ACTUALLY THE NORM

Health providers, physicians, and nurses refer a woman to a radiologic facility for screening mammography. Mammography is divided arbitrary and artificially in two parts. One is called screening mammography and the other diagnostic mammography (a misnomer). We should mention that mammography cannot make a diagnosis of breast cancer. Diagnosis of breast cancer is made only on the specimen of the lesion by pathologists. Screening mammography is done for patients who have no symptoms, presumed normal despite the fact that we know breast cancer at the beginning has no symptoms. Diagnostic mammography is done for patients who have symptoms such as mass in the breast or abnormality seen on the screening mammography. It consists of taking more pictures (spot, magnification) of the abnormality for further evaluation.

For screening mammography, at a radiologic facility the patient gets two pictures from each breast by an x-ray technologist and leaves the facility without seeing or being examined by any physician or specialist. If the patient has a question, no answer can be provided. The patient has to wait anxiously ten to fifteen days until her health provider informs her of the results. If the patient needs more tests or extra imaging views, she should come back. That is the beginning of inconveniences. In this second radiology visit, if the patient still needs more tests, such as MRI, ultrasound, core biopsy, the patient has to wait again until being informed by her referring physician or referring health provider, and for this test an authorization from the insurance company is necessary. Once it is obtained, sometimes the radiologic facility does not have the appropriate means for diagnosis such as core needle biopsy under the control of ultrasonography or MRI, and the patient should go elsewhere to a more specialized facility called breast imaging center, which is not located in every corner, many times far distant from the patient's residence.

Once the diagnosis of breast cancer is made, for surgery, the patient has to go to a different place which often duplicates previous tests. After surgery, the patient is referred to an oncologist or radiotherapist all at different sites. Sometimes, this back-and-forth diagnostic tests and treatments may take months. By that time, cancer may progress much further and the treatment delayed. It seems that this policy was adopted because of economical reason (gatekeeper policy). If it is so, this is precisely a pure miscalculation (pennywise pound foolish). Because no referral physician ever denies extra tests requested by the radiologist, particularly in the matter of breast cancer. This policy leads to enormous discomfort for the patient, especially in elderlies. A big hassle, paperwork, and telephone calls between the referring health provider and radiologist become more costly for the patient and insurance companies, and most important, it delays the treatment of breast cancer. The comprehensive breast center teamwork in Van Nuys (California) proved its validity in better medical care and more cost-effectiveness for the patient and society.

There is no doubt that for eye problem or heart disease, it is much better to see a specialist than a general practitioner or other health provider. Nonetheless, there are certain minor problems that can be managed by a general practitioner before seeing a specialist. This differs in the matter of the breast. The whole purpose of medical visit of the patient is to detect her breast cancer at the earliest stage. Early breast cancer has no sign, neither objective nor subjective. It can be detected only by mammography, ultrasonography, MRI, or core needle biopsy. None of them is in the domain of any general practitioner. Another problem is that with the new legislation, radiologists should inform a patient as well as her physician of the status of the patient's breast density. High-dense breasts are considered as a high risk for breast cancer. Neither the patient nor her physician knows what to do or what measure to be taken as an extra step. This is because of lack of guidelines. A gynecologist colleague told me that in order to avoid any liability, he will order MRI and ultrasonography to any dense breast. Imagine the cost of such a policy. All these types of problems can be resolved conveniently in a comprehensive breast center; our guideline is described in chapter 17.

A comprehensive breast center has the following advantages:

1. Direct visit of the patient for screening breast cancer or any other problem, high-degree of patient satisfaction, no waste of time. Screening breast cancer requires the availability of the physical examination, screening mammography, ultrasonography, and MRI.
2. Most efficient way for rapid and early breast cancer detection without delay for the treatment. Detection, diagnosis, treatment of breast cancer, and follow-up of patients all done in one place.
3. Most efficient way economically for the patient and society (for insurance companies).
4. Most efficient way in contributing to the progress of breast cancer knowledge, working under one roof with all breast specialties.

In conclusion, we are spending millions of dollars in searching and studying to find ways to improve our health care in terms of quality and cost. Comprehensive breast center is one example where the finish study is already done; it suffices to duplicate it in large scale.

STRUCTURE OF THE COMPREHENSIVE BREAST CENTER

The structure of the comprehensive breast center is composed of a surgical oncologist, medical oncologist, plastic surgeon, radiologist, radiotherapist, pathologist, psychologist, geneticist, nutritionist.

The majority of the public does not know the role of each specialist in breast cancer. We explain briefly their work.

The role of the surgeon in the comprehensive breast center: The role of the surgeon is very important because patients follow the advice of their surgeon in submitting themselves to any kind of surgery that the surgeon suggests. Skill in surgery and deep knowledge of breast imaging play a great role in complete eradication of breast cancer with a good cosmetic result and preservation of the breast. The more conservative the surgeon, the better for the patient, and it's less costly for the society.

The role of the medical oncologist in the comprehensive breast center: A medical oncologist is an internist specializing in medical treatment of cancer, some of whom are more experienced and more specialized in the treatment of breast cancer. Experience and knowledge of the medical oncologist in the matter of new techniques, MRI, PET/CT scan, and genetic tests and interpretation of laboratory tests lead to better, more efficient treatment of breast cancer. Chemotherapy causes numerous damages, sometimes worse than the cancer itself. Chemotherapy has created another branch of medicine to treat the damage of the side effects of toxic medication of chemotherapy. Thus the supervision of the oncologist during and following the treatment of breast cancer is indispensable.

The role of plastic surgeon in the comprehensive breast center: The plastic surgeon plays a great role in the life of breast cancer patients. Losing a breast by mastectomy or deformity of the breast after surgery is psychologically stressful and is a great issue particularly for the young female. Plastic surgery can be a savior to revive the spirit of the breast cancer patient.

The role of radiologist in the comprehensive breast center: A large number of people do not know that the radiologist is a medical doctor with five or more years of training in the science of radiology. Because the radiologist in the USA has no contact with patients, they are not recognized by the public as a medical doctor. The American College of Radiology in the last ten years has attempted to make known the real face of the radiologist to the public without any success. The public recognizes someone as a medical doctor who takes care of patients. It should be known that radiologists specializing in breast imaging carry the greatest role in the management of breast cancer. Their role consists of detection of early breast cancer as well as detection of metastasis. These radiologists specialize in many fields such as interpreting mammography, ultrasonography, breast MRI, nuclear medicine, and PET scan. The decision taken by other colleagues for the management of breast cancer depends greatly on the report of the radiologist. Radiologists perform procedures such as ductography, fine needle aspiration cytology, punch biopsy, core needle biopsy by stereotactic or under the control of ultrasonography or MRI, preoperative needle localization of the lesion for the surgeon, and injection of radioisotope into the breast for localization of axillary sentinel lymph node biopsy, and finally follow up patient after the treatment of breast cancer by the same protocol. The success in the treatment of breast cancer depends largely on the skill and experience of the radiologist.

The role of the radiotherapist or radiation oncologist in the comprehensive breast center: The radiation oncologist is a medical doctor, trained and specializing in radiation therapy of all types of cancer, and with cooperation of radiation physicist, determines the ports (entrance of radiation), the dose and the sequences and duration of radiation therapy follow-up of the patient during treatment. Radiation oncologist treats also the complications and side effects of irradiated breast.

The role of the pathologist in the comprehensive breast center: The pathologist is a medical doctor trained and specializing in pathology (macroscopic and microscopic and histochemistry of cancer). Modality of the treatment of breast cancer depends on the pathologic findings. The pathologist makes the diagnosis of cancer and also determines the nature and the degree of aggressiveness by measuring the size and histochemistry of breast cancer. Expertise of pathologist in the matter of breast cancer is of paramount importance. Misinterpretation leads to irreparable damage.

The role of the psychologist in the comprehensive breast center: The psycho-oncologist, either a physician psychiatrist or the psychologist with experience in matters of breast cancer, also plays a great role in the treatment of breast cancer. "Treat the mind before the body" was the motto of Dr. Charles Gros. Disclosure of bad news of breast cancer to the patient is a great shock. A patient with high degree of anxiety and desperation in acute state of depression may attempt irrational decision or suicide. On the other hand, even when the patient overcomes the acute phase of depression, sometimes chronic depression continues, due to therapy, surgery, radiotherapy, and chemotherapy. Psychological consultation and support can restore hope and good morale to the patient. It is unfortunate that often psychology consultation is forgotten and patients continue to suffer from chronic anxieties or depression.

The role of the geneticist in the comprehensive breast center: Genetic counseling is important for patients who have family history of breast or ovarian cancer, particularly patients who have been found with damaged genes BRC1 and BRC2. Those patients need genetic counseling for thorough explanation of appropriate treatment for herself and her family.

The role of the nutritionist in the comprehensive breast center: A patient with breast cancer is traumatized in her mind and body and may get worse after surgery and radiation therapy, particularly during chemotherapy and hormone therapy. Side effects of these therapies may cause loss of energy, appetite, vomiting, hypotension, and loss or gain of weight. Therefore, a correct and calculated nutrition, adequate fluid intake, correct amount of vitamins and minerals should be instituted. Appropriate nutrition is the key for health. It is well known that malnutrition diminishes immunity of the body, exposing the patient to a variety of illnesses, lowers resistance to infection, and favors progression of cancer. In this regard, a nutritionist is of great value. The role of the social worker is very important and not enough emphasized in long-term care of patients with terminal illness.

STANDARDS AND STATISTICS IN MEDICINE

STANDARDS

In this book we will be talking in many instances of standards in breast cancer management. But what is the standard in medicine?

Standard is a setup of strict rules decreed by official authorities as a model to be followed by practitioners. Standards can be imposed particularly to all types of industries—car industries, food industries, building industries, health hazard industries, and pharmaceutical industries, all for the protection of the consumer. In general, standards in these industries work because all elements are known; it suffices to put all together and make a necessary rule.

In medicine, a science of uncertainty, majority of biological elements are unknown. They change every instant, and every day new elements are discovered. Modern medicine on its best day is a very complex brew, not lending itself to rigid rule imposed by a standard. In medicine, nothing is permanent except changes. Imposing standards in medicine is a good procedure, but it should be commensurate with the progress of technology. A pretty standard procedure of today may turn ugly tomorrow.

For a hundred years, radical mastectomy, removal of the breast, chest wall muscles, and lymph node dissection were the standards of operable breast cancer treatment. Any deviation of those standards was considered criminal. Today, new standard of treatment of early breast cancer is the preservation of the breast, radiation; and if axillary lymph node positive, then chemotherapy. Again, deviation from this new standard in medicine is a liability even if done in the interest of the patient. In the court of law, deviation from the standard is not defensible. That is why all patients with breast cancer receive the same treatment (one size fits all), which is a clear overtreatment for some patients. Standards in medicine take time to be changed. There have always been heroic efforts of some brilliant minds to deviate from the standards such as Barnard in South Africa for heart transplant, without him, we would still not have practicing heart transplants, for saving thousands of lives. Fisher in the USA, by randomized trials, showed that mastectomy and preservation of the breast have the same result of survival, without him, radical mastectomy would still have been practiced all over the world for small operable breast cancers. Ligos in San Francisco pioneered and showed that DCIS can be treated without radiation. Deviation from standards in medicine is very dangerous in the beginning, but if it turns to be successful, then it becomes standard.

STATISTICS

Medicine is a matter of balancing risks and benefits. Statistics is very important for us because all our actions, particularly in breast cancer, are based on statistics.

Statistics may be the result of inadequate research. A bad research is worse than no research. Incorrect conclusion may cause irreparable harm. Treatment of breast cancer is based statistically on the result of prospective randomized trial. However, there is no guarantee that the result of trials is meaningful. Statistically "significant" does not always equal to clinical significance. Statistical significance by itself is not necessarily a proof that the hypothesis is correct. The secret language of statistics is appealing that one can easily manipulate, inflate, sensationalize, or oversimplify the data. In practice the data may not fulfill any shining promise of statistics. In the *New England Journal of Medicine*, in reviewing sixty-three medical articles between 1995 and 1997 on statistics errors, it was found that 48% of articles had mistakes in how they calculated. There are always flaws in any large medical study particularly in clinical randomized trials, especially if the study is performed through a large number of centers. There have been gross comments about statistics. One published booklet was titled *How to Lie With Statistics* (D. Huff) ("lies, damned lies, statistics" [Disraeli]). Published medical statistics is very useful, but it should be taken into account with great caution.

TERM OF RISK USED IN BREAST CANCER

Two terms—one is absolute risk and the other relative risk—are used in breast cancer. They can be confusing if not given a clear explanation.

Absolute risk: A young girl without family history asks her physician, "What is my lifetime risk of breast cancer?" The physician responds, "12%" (about 1 out of 8 females). This is absolute risk.

Relative risk: It is always evaluated by comparison. For example, a number of patients with the same baseline risk (e.g., 4%) of breast cancer. Patients are divided into two groups. One group is given experimental medication for reducing breast cancer. Nothing is given to the second group (placebo). We look at the result after five years. In the group that received the medication, cancer was reduced to 3%. Here the difference is 1% (absolute risk), but one is one-fourth of the four, which makes 25%. This is relative risk reduction. This is often used by physicians who want to magnify the efficacy of their medication. If you tell the patient that a medication which causes side effects reduces only 1% your risk of cancer, most likely the patient will refuse to take the medication. But if you tell her that the medication reduces 25% the risk of cancer, the patient may accept voluntarily the medication despite its serious side effects.

Another relative risk: Two groups are again used. In one group the baseline risk of breast cancer is 3 per thousand. After five years of medication, the risk was reduced to 1 per thousand; relative risk reduction is 300%. In the other group, the baseline risk of breast cancer is 3 per million. After five years, the risk is reduced to 1 in a million. Relative risk reduction is still 300%. In these two experiments, in the first group, 2 per thousand patients get the benefit of medication, and in one million makes two thousand patients. Therefore the medication is indicated in the first group, because in the second group, only two patients in one million benefited from the medication; therefore, the medication is not indicated despite the fact that the relative risk for both was 300%. In conclusion, the patients should know that absolute risk is important, not the relative risk. And we as physicians should always tell them the absolute figure of the benefit or the risk of our intervention and procedures.

CHAPTER 2

BRIEF ANATOMY AND PHYSIOLOGY OF THE BREAST

The internal structure of the breast is composed of eight different elements important in breast cancer.

1. Milk glands: Provide milk, steroid hormones, growth hormone, immunoglobulin, and numerous proteinase. Milk glands in pregnancy look like a grapevine; otherwise, they look like a winter tree (fig. 8.13). Its trunk opens to the nipple. Branches divide to narrow ducts, ductules, and end up to the numerous cul-de-sacs called lobules. Each tree occupies a territory called lobe; each breast has one to twenty lobes. Each lobe can independently be involved with different benign type of lesions, such as ductectasia, papilloma, adenoma, or malignancy.
2. Myoepithelial cells: These are small muscular cells surrounding the milk ducts. Their contraction propels milk to the nipple.
3. Fibroblastic cells surrounding the milk duct: Their role is as supportive tissue. In breast cancer, there is constant communication, talking between fibroblastic cells and cancerous epithelial cells. Fibroblastic cells react against stress, forming a barrier of fibrocystic scar, and are the origin of fibrosarcoma.
4. Collagenous proteinous material: This is a proteinous material, semifluid embedding all the breast structures.

5. Fatty tissue: Source of steroid hormones interposed between the milk glands. It is the origin of liposarcoma.
6. Arteries: Channels carrying oxygen, blood, and nutrients to the breast tissue. They are the origin of angiosarcoma.
7. Veins: Channels returning deoxygenated blood to the heart and vehiculing breast cancer metastasis to the heart.
8. Lymphatic system: Carries essentially metabolic waste and also metastatic cells to the heart then from the heart via arteries to the rest of the body. It is the origin of lymphoma and lymphosarcoma.

The picture shows that metastasis from breast cancer can be transported directly to the lymph nodes in the axilla, neck, behind the sternum, and to the opposite breast and axilla, interconnection with abdominal lymphatic channels to visceral organs.

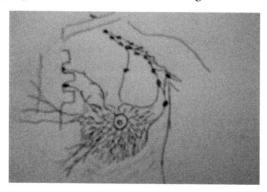

BRIEF PHYSIOLOGY OF THE BREAST

The breast physiology, interactions, and interdependences with other secretory structures of the body, such as hypothalamus, pituitary gland, adrenal glands, thyroid glands, and ovarian glands, are highly complex. We are interested only in clinical repercussion of the physiological changes of breast function. Each organ has its circadian clock which may influence its requirement for the treatment. Hormone fluctuation in premenopausal period has great importance in the detection and treatment of breast cancer. As a female approaches her menstrual cycle, hormonal change increases. Hemodynamic pressure in the breast mainly in the third week of the cycle rises. The breast vessels become engorged and congested; the breasts become larger, tender, painful, and sensitive. Metabolism in the breast increases. The breast temperature hikes, emanating more infrared rays. This can be seen by electronic thermography. All these phenomena recess after the menstrual cycle.

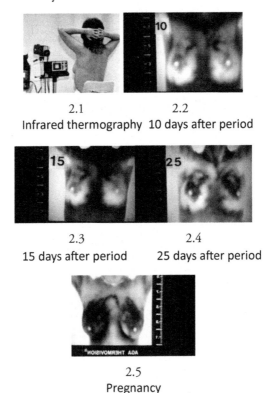

2.1   2.2
Infrared thermography 10 days after period

2.3   2.4
15 days after period   25 days after period

2.5
Pregnancy

Notice the connection of blood vessels of two breasts. Cancer cells can migrate easily from one to other breast and other parts of the body. Engorgement of breast shown in fifteenth and twenty-fifth days after period and during pregnancy.

We learn the following from this observation of normal physiology of the breast:

1. Self-examination or physical examination by the health provider should be done regularly in the second weeks after the menstrual cycle; otherwise, bumpy/lumpy congestive breast at palpation may lead to other useless tests.

2. Mammography should be done in the first two weeks post-menstrual cycle. If mammography is done at the third week, the breast may be very sensitive and painful because of congestion. Images of breast tissue may be denser with ill-defined densities indistinguishable with abnormal lesion requiring more useless tests.

3. MRI should be done in the first two weeks after the menstrual cycle. If the patient takes hormones, they should be stopped for two weeks in order to avoid false positive image due to hormonal angiogenesis, which can cause white foci suspicious for malignancy and useless biopsy performed.

4. Surgery of the breast should be done in the first two weeks after the menstrual cycle to avoid bleeding and late healing and eventually to prevent release of cancerous cells and their migrations.

TOPOGRAPHY OF THE BREAST

How do we localize breast cancer clinically and radiologically? In order to determine the site of cancer, we divide the breast in four quadrants: upper outer quadrant, lower outer quadrant, upper inner quadrant, and lower inner quadrant.

Example: Left breast

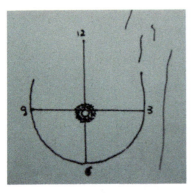

12 to 3 o'clock upper outer quadrant

3 to 6 o'clock outer lower quadrant

6 to 9 o'clock lower inner quadrant

9 to 12 o'clock upper inner quadrant

2.6

This is how we indicate medically right and left side of the breasts as we look at the patient standing in front of us.

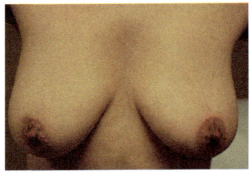

2.7

CHAPTER 3

HOW CANCER IS BORN

BRIEF MOLECULAR GENESIS OF BREAST CANCER

Our body is composed of approximately one hundred trillion cells. Each cell normally has forty-six (germ cell 23) chromosomes except for red cells. The chromosomes are composed of double helix of DNA. DNA is composed of about twenty-five thousand genes with 10 million protein and 6 billion bases. Genes carry predetermined mission for formation of organs and their function. Cells function normally as long as there is a balance between function of different proteins. In each cell, there is a nucleus, which is the black box of the cell and contains protein called proto-oncogene or precancerous material, and under certain circumstances mutation takes place. Mutation is the change in sequences of protein which may promote proto-oncogene to oncogene (formation of cancer). There are also in each cell other proteins such as BRC1, BRC2, and P53, called tumor suppressors. Their mission is to prevent the promotion of proto-oncogene to oncogene. These genes have also the function to repair if there is damage in the chromosomes.

Our cells are under constant attack by germs, bacteria, viruses, bugs, x-rays, gamma rays, chemo toxins, and traumas, which can harm the DNA and promote cancer. These damages can cause deletion, breakage, aneuploidy trisomia of chromosomes, and in molecular level, damage to the DNA, and displacement of the protein can repress or inactivate the function of cells. When a DNA gene duplicates, it is called overamplification. It also causes the increase of oncogenic protein on the surface of the cells, called overexpression. In hereditary breast cancer, mainly two genes, BRC1 and BRC2, and in sporadic breast cancer non-hereditary more than two hundred genes have been implicated. Another hypothetical thesis put forward in the genesis of cancer formation is that cancer can be produced without genetic mutation, without change in the sequence of the gene, but only by alteration of gene expression, called epigenetic process. This mechanism of action can be reversible; thus one day, we probably would be able to turn on and turn off the genesis of breast cancer.

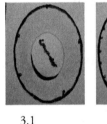

3.1 Normal cells

3.2 Cancer cell, duplication of chromosome, and increased abnormal proteins at cell's surface

ANATOMIC GENESIS OF BREAST CANCER

About 85% of breast cancer originates from the cells of milk glands. Milk glands are composed of ducts and lobules. Breast cancer that develops in the duct is called ductal carcinoma in situ (DCIS). Overdevelopment of the cells in the lobule is called lobular carcinoma in situ (LCIS). Invasive cancer originating from the duct is called invasive ductal carcinoma. Invasive cancer developing from lobules is called invasive lobular carcinoma. DCIS has a 40% propensity to turn into invasive carcinoma. LCIS is considered as a high risk for development of breast cancer on either side. Breast cancer can be originated from a few milk ducts (focally) or from a large number of milk ducts (segmentally) or from the entire milk ducts of the breast (globally).

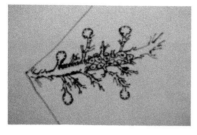 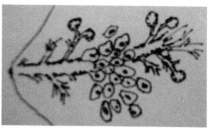

3.3
Cancer cells inside of the duct, DCIS; morphology, noninvasive

3.4
Cancer cells rupturing ductal wall and spreading in the breast; morphology, invasive cancer

Thus, when cancer develops in the breast, it causes intense turbulence in the entire structure of the breast.

1. Breast cancer cells are extremely avid of the blood supply and need sugar, more oxygen, minerals, hormones, and proteins for fast proliferation. In order to sustain their rapid development they secrete chemical substances with specific function; one of them, and most important, is the angiogenic factor, which dilates more active blood vessels, reactivates dormant vessels, and forms new vessels (called neoangiogenesis). As cancer grows, for more rapid blood exchange, it forms arteriovenous shunt inside and outside of the tumor mass. It has been well demonstrated in laboratory animals. In humans, breast cancer tumor deviates all blood vessels and blood supply of the chest wall toward itself, causing ischemia of the opposite side, well demonstrated by MRI and also thermography. Neoangiogenesis is formed by irregular-shaped and fast-growing vascular endothelial cells; in laboratory, they survive three to four days, whereas normal cells live only one day. No basement membrane exists in neoangiogenesis; endothelial cells are distant from each other; that is why the vessel leaks.

2. High cellular metabolism of cancer increases the temperature of the involved breast (breast fever), which can be

demonstrated by electronic thermography. Sometimes the level of temperature could reach 40°C. A veritable furnace in the cells.

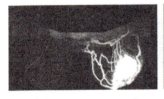 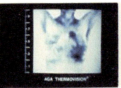

Right   3.5   Left

On MRI, all blood flow deviated toward the cancer mass on the left side, no blood supply for the right.

Right   Left   3.6   Right   Left

Thermography: Breast cancer can be detected by its heat, fever of the breast; higher metabolism in cancer tissue increases infrared rays by which we detect cancer; again all blood of chest wall pooled on the left-side breast cancer. In color picture, breast cancer and its intramammary lymph node metastasis are white, meaning 5 centigrade higher in temperature of the lesion.

Left

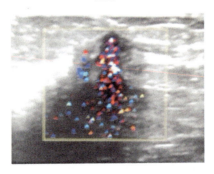

3.7

Ultrasound: The dark image is consistent with invasive cancer and vascularity is demonstrated by Doppler technique by the red color.

Right	Left	Left side magnification

3.8   3.9

Mammography: On the left side, large calcified nutrient artery (*arrow*) circles the mass of cancer, and its branches converge to the center of cancerous tissue.

We stress very much on breast cancer angiogenesis. The reason is that formation of new vessels by cancer cells supply more food for development of cancer, and by stopping the formation of vessels, we can bring cancer cells to death. That's what we do now through genetic war, targeting specific protein promoter of angiogenesis by destroying them with chemical bullets. By cutting food supply, we may get long remission and eventually cure.

1. Disturbance of the blood circulation causes hemodynamic changes in the breast. It increases hydrostatic pressure in the interstitial fluid and lymphatic system, leading to diffuse edema of the breast, which can be seen even in DCIS and can be demonstrated by mammography.
2. Cancer cells can form new milk ducts, called neoductogenisis, either by reactivating dehiscent milk ducts or forming new ducts (fig. 3.10). Exceptionally permeable, which can be demonstrated by a ductogram.

3. Cancer cells during their development inflame the rest of the breast structure, increasing the density of the breast by provoking collagenic protein, called collagenosis, and increasing fibroblastic reaction, called fibrosis, causing dimpling, retraction, and contraction of the breast. These can be seen by mammography and physical examination.
4. Proliferation and hypertrophy of the fatty breast tissue (lipocytes) around cancer mass, which can be demonstrated only by mammography and histology and felt by clinical examination, reported as a peritumoral lipogenesis. The significance of this phenomenon is unknown; defensive reaction? This type of cancer is usually highly estrogen receptor positive, good prognosis.

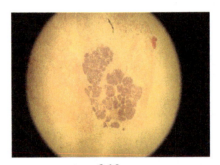

3.10
Histology
Microscopic image, neoductogenesis (new formation of duct) stands out in darker color.

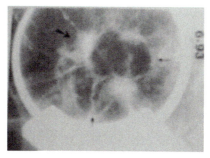

3.11
Xray(spot)
Peritumoral lipogenesis cancer image is in white (1.5 cm); fat is in black. This is a cancer of the soft consistency which can be taken for breast lipoma on physical examination

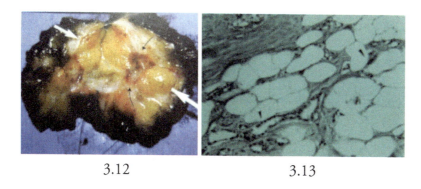

3.12   3.13

(Fig. 3.11) This patient came for a soft tissue mass of more than 6 cm in diameter in her left breast with diagnosis of large lipoma (fatty tumor), spot magnified. Mammography shows well small spiculated mass surrounded by large fatty compartments. Resection of the entire mass (fig. 3.12) shows small cancer of 1.5 cm (*black fine arrows*) and surrounded by large yellow fatty masses (*white arrows*). Microscopic examination showed large fatty cells in white (fig. 3.13). This is a cancer of soft consistency which can be taken on physical examination for breast lipoma as was in this case. It is very important for the clinician to be aware of such an entity so as not to be misled.

CONCLUSION

The knowledge of all anatomic changes in the breast caused by cancer is very important for detection of breast cancer on mammography.

Some changes called direct sign of breast cancer demonstrated on mammography as mass density or microcalcifications; other six changes that we described constitute indirect signs of breast cancer. All of the above changes can be seen all together at once on screening mammography reported for the first time in author's book *Atlas of Mammography* (1996).

CHAPTER 4

HOW BREAST CANCER DEVELOPS AND SPREADS METASTASIS

BIOLOGY OF BREAST CANCER

Genetically mutated milk breast cells may transform to cancerous lesions. Cancerous cells become autonomous, totally out of our body's control. Cancerous cells inherit all the characteristics of normal cells such as reproduction, secretion of hormones, metabolic function, etc. In addition, in their new factories, they can fabricate a new material that were not produced in normal milk cells, such as production of bone and cartilage (producing osteosarcoma or osteochondroma).

Theoretically, cancer cells by anarchic cloning can give birth to an immortal monster in our body. Fortunately it doesn't. Breast cancer is a criminal that does not obey any rules. Its natural history is unpredictable. Histologically, it is postulated that mutated cells first become atypical cells, slightly larger than normal duct cells. The second step is the transformation to ductal carcinoma in situ. The cells are still larger, more irregular, and multilayered, confined inside the duct. About 40% of DCIS is transformed to invasive breast carcinoma (Page D., pathologist). By rupturing the ductal wall, they become invasive. The frontier between ductal carcinoma in situ and invasive cancer is just the presence of the ductal wall. This is an anatomical border but not a biological frontier. DCIS cells get the mission of invasiveness before rupturing the ductal walls. It is postulated that when DCIS transforms to invasive carcinoma, it secretes different substances such as angiogenic factors (vascular endothelial growth factor), bradykinin, prostaglandin, and nitric oxide; all contribute to the spread of metastasis and to hyperpermeability of the tumor cells for further nutrition.

Pathologic evolution of breast cancer
Classic notion

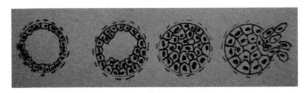

4.1
Normal duct   hyperplasia   DCIS   invasive

Mammographic evolution of breast cancer

1983 DCIS not detected   1988 invasive cancer

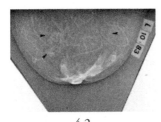 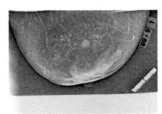

4.2   4.3
Neoductogenesis DCIS (arrows)   DCIS + invasive cancer

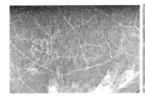 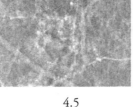 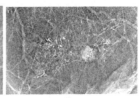

4.4   4.5   4.6

Magnification of above picture cluster of neoductogenesis white tortuous tubes DCIS

Spot film of tortuous ducts

Microcalcifications DCIS (white particles) & round white nodule invasive breast cancer

1. MECHANISM OF GENETIC METASTASIS

Recent genetic discovery in breast cancer challenges the classical notion of breast cancer formation, which assumes that sequential evolution of the ductal mutated cells leads to ductal hyperplasia, then to DCIS, DCIS to invasive breast cancer tumor, then to metastasis, arguing that the ability of spreading metastasis is not during the formation of the tumor but it is a genetic property. That means that the mission of metastatogenecity is established in molecular stage long before we detect cancer mass. Thus different types of mutation in the DNA chain can cause different entities, benign or malignant. All cancer cells with different missions, with different outcomes, look alike under the microscope. But genetic tests differentiate good cancer from the bad cancer, high risk from the low risk for metastasis. That means that cancer that by morphology looks benign, like DCIS, can spread metastasis; it is not necessary for DCIS to transform morphologically to invasive to spread metastasis.

Mutation in normal milk cells may progress to hyperplasia without further changes or to DCIS without further progress, or to DCIS with mission of metastasis without rupturing ductal walls, or progresses to invasive by rupturing ductal walls and metastasis. Independent genetic transformations from normal duct are shown below.

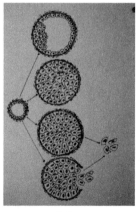

Hyperplasia

DCIS no metastatic mission

DCIS with metastatic mission without rupturing ductal wall Metastasis

DCIS with mission to invasive cancer with metastasis, rupturing the duct wall

4.6

Metastasis is the migration of cancer cells from breast cancer to other organs via lymphovascular channels. Clinically, to detect breast cancer metastasis is to find cancerous cells in the axillae by surgical lymph node sampling. Recent genetic study of breast cancer has shown that once angiogenesis is formed, metastatic cells selectively can get access either to the lymphatic channels (lymphogenic metastasis) or to the blood vessels (hematogenic metastasis). Contrary to the old belief, there is no relation between the two of them. A patient may have distant metastasis without lymph node involvement or vice versa. Distal metastasis is due to hematogenic spread. Cancer cells with metastatic mission separate from primary tumor mass and enter the blood vessels, and after a period of time, cancer cells exit from the blood circulation and graft on a selected organ (soil and seed). If the organ accepts the implant, cancer cells proliferate and form an angiogenic network, and metastasis is organized. Appropriateness of soil contributes to the survival of the metastasis.

Progression of the metastasis depends on genetic signature of the primary breast cancer. If primary is a highly aggressive metastasis carrying the same character. It should be mentioned that metastatic cells are navigated by specific proteins in each step of their journey, entering the blood circulation, exiting from it, grafting on the selected organ, and progressing and invading the organ. The question arises, how can proteins accomplish all this sophisticated and complicated functions?

2. INTRADUCTAL CARCINOMA IN SITU IS A CANCER?

All epithelial breast cancer in the beginning is in situ (DCIS). Of hundreds of breast cancers that we detect today, 25% of them are DCIS and 75% are invasive breast cancer. Of the 25% DCIS, 95% of them are detected by mammography because of microcalcifications, and 5% by mass formation (tumor). Biologic characteristics of this detectable DCIS are well studied. DCIS with microcalcification has 50% propensity to invasive cancer. 75% of breast cancer that we detect are invasive, but one day, all these cancers were in situ, undetectable (no microcalcifications). Therefore, we do not have any clue of their biology, certainly different with those ones we detect with microcalcifications.

Ductal carcinoma in situ is called noninvasive breast cancer because some physicians believe that DCIS is not a cancer; some others call it precancerous lesions. There are proofs that some DCIS have all quiescent criteria of a forthright invasive cancer: genetic similarity, proclivity to invasion, spreading metastasis, causing death.

DOES DCIS METASTASIZE?

It is postulated that metastasis is a function of invasive breast cancer. However, 2% to 7% lymph node metastasis and 2% mortality in DCIS have been reported in medical literature. More interesting is that in those mastectomies, no invasive carcinoma has been found. The notion of invasiveness and noninvasiveness is based on pathologic observation of the integrity of the ductal wall. Today, with genetic discovery, that notion is obsolete because DCIS with intact ducts can be aggressive and can metastasize without rupturing the ductal walls. It is conceived that DCIS with aggressive mission secretes a lytic enzyme that dissolves ductal wall and basement membrane, and the cancer cells exit the ducts and continue their proliferation and infiltrate the periductal tissue and secrete angiogenic factors by which it can spread their metastasis. **It should be mentioned that if DCIS cells do not get the mission of invasiveness, they would not secrete any lytic enzymes nor rupture ductal wall and would not infiltrate outside the wall; they would remain permanently inside the duct.**

A. METASTASIS OF DCIS WITHOUT RUPTURING DUCTAL WALLS

Electronic microscopy shows that there are tiny spaces between ductal cells; mutated cancer cells with mission of aggressiveness decreasing gap junction protein then by amoeboid movement can pass through these spaces without destroying the walls, getting out of the duct and forming angiogenesis and spreading the metastasis.

We had several cases of DCIS with very aggressive nature called killer DCIS, an entity detected by mammography manifested by specific type of microcalcification, crushed-stone or road-like branching linear microcalcification, high-grade lesion pathologically with intact ductal wall. One fatal case reported in 1996 in the author's book that DCIS with intact ducts in fact was invasive breast cancer in the cloth of noninvasive lesion.

In August 1983, thirty-eight-year-old patient felt a palpable mass in her right breast. Mammography showed broken stone-like calcifications of the mass. Biopsy showed 2.5 cm DCIS. The patient underwent lumpectomy and breast irradiation. In 1985, local recurrence with calcifications, biopsy showed 2.5 cm comedo DCIS with macroinvasion. The patient underwent mastectomy and breast reconstruction.

In October 1986, chest wall invasive recurrence occurred and six months later died of general metastasis.

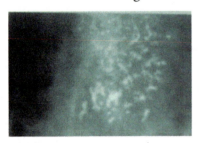

This picture shows clustered crushed stone-type of microcalcifications due to the intense necrosis of dead cells typical for killer DCIS.

4.7

Typical evolution of the killer DCIS: first DCIS, second invasive recurrence, third chest wall invasion, fourth general metastasis and demise—all 3.5 years duration, most likely metastasis has been spread in 1983 before morphologic transformation of DCIS to microinvasion in 1985.

In this case it can be argued that if the patient had mastectomy at the onset of DCIS diagnosis, it would have prevented invasive occurrence and would have changed the outcome; it would be valid if we accept that metastasis takes place only in invasive phase of cancer. But if metastasis spreads in DCIS stage, mastectomy would not have any effect on the outcome. However, in this type of DCIS after diagnosis by mammography signs and histology grade III, oncotype Dx > 55 mastectomy may eventually provide a better chance of survival. Chemotherapy is not the standard of practice in DCIS, but in this type of DCIS it would be most likely beneficial.

B. METASTASIS OF DCIS WITHOUT RUPTURING THE DUCTAL WALLS BUT BY FORMATION OF ENDODUCTAL ANGIOGENESIS

Histologic demonstration of extraductal neoangiogenesis has been reported in literature, but intraductal angiogenesis formation of the vessel <u>inside the duct</u> was shown for the first time by the author in 1996 and in 1998 in Dr. Mel Silverstein's book (chapter 5).

In fact, DCIS cells with mission of aggressiveness are capable of forming angiogenesis inside the duct, which communicates with the vessels outside the duct. Cancer cells can metastasize through intraductal vessels without destroying or rupturing the ductal wall. That is how we demonstrated in the following case. In 1990, we were interested in the subject of breast cancer angiogenesis because at that time many publications reported that invasive breast cancer with more angiogenesis had the worst prognosis. Thus, we wanted to know if that notion was valid in DCIS. We requested our pathologists to perform immunostaining of our DCIS with factor IV; surprisingly, pathologists found two cases of intraductal angiogenesis inside the duct with intact walls. We present here the case that we have meticulously followed up.

HISTORY OF A FIFTY-TWO-YEAR-OLD POST-MENOPAUSAL WOMAN. Her mammography showed fatty breast with a small dense nodule in the inner side of the right breast. By bracketing hook-wire localization, a mass of 7 mm DCIS with more than 1 cm clear margin was removed. Immunostaining showed endoductal angiogenesis (fig. 4.10). The patient had radiation followed by regular checkup every six months. In the third year, mammography showed no breast recurrence but developed distant metastasis. That proves that most likely metastases have been spread in DCIS stage.

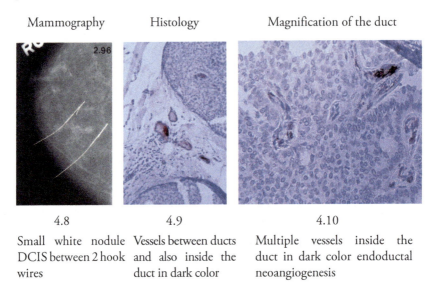

Mammography	Histology	Magnification of the duct
4.8	4.9	4.10
Small white nodule DCIS between 2 hook wires	Vessels between ducts and also inside the duct in dark color	Multiple vessels inside the duct in dark color endoductal neoangiogenesis

THE END OF NATURAL HISTORY OF SOME INVASIVE BREAST CANCER

Certain DCIS never turn to invasive cancer. Some invasive breast cancer never manifests clinically. Others never metastasize. These conditions can be found at the time of autopsy. About 58% of patients die of invasive breast cancer in two circumstances.

1. Local breast cancer invasion
2. Distant organ metastasis

<u>Local breast invasion</u>. Today, this is rare in Western countries but in the past was more common. Breast cancer if not treated gradually progresses, opens to the skin and burgeons, ulcerating, bleeding, getting bacterial and fungal infection, ending to malodorous putrefaction, and finally systemic intractable fever and death. Another form of local invasion is that with breast cancer treated by mastectomy with

or without radiation therapy, small subcutaneous nodules appear on the chest wall and at the site of mastectomy, gradually ulcerating and finally ending up with the same outcome as the previous case.

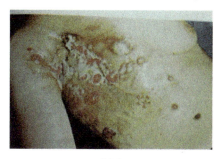

4.11

Chest wall recurrence, ulcerations post-mastectomy and radiation therapy

<u>Distant organ metastasis</u>. Finding of distant organ metastasis is more common today, cancer metastasis invading and destroying vital organs such as brain, lung, liver, and viscera, causing death of the patient. For that, there is a race between distant metastasis and local chest wall invasion.

CONCLUSION:

The most important fact for us is to detect breast cancer in its DCIS state, because the chance of definitive cure lies there.

Metastasis is determinant factor of the patient's outcome.

Metastasis ability is a genetic property before formation of cancerous mass.

Genetic test determines the risk of metastasis, better than microscopic histology of cancer.

Endoneoangiogenesis in DCIS is a high risk for metastasis.

If immunostaining were carried out routinely in DCIS, it would have changed dramatically its treatment.

CHAPTER 5

BILATERALITY OF BREAST CANCER

The breasts are excellent organs to give birth to cancer. Patients who catch breast cancer in one breast are at high risk to develop cancer in the opposite breast, contralateral breast. If both cancers are detected at the same time, it is called synchronous; if the second cancer is detected later, it is called metachronous cancer. In the olden days, about 25% of cancers were discovered simultaneously, and 75% were detected metachronously. It was also postulated that cancer diagnosed clinically simultaneously were the worse prognosis than metachronous cancer. The longer space between the occurrence of the second cancer in the opposite side, the better the prognosis.

High risks for bilaterality of breast cancer:

1. A patient diagnosed with one-sided breast cancer is at higher risk to develop breast cancer on the opposite side.
2. Age: A patient with more advanced age with one-sided breast cancer is at higher risk of bilaterality.
3. A patient with one-sided breast cancer with a strong family history of breast carcinoma is at increased risk of bilaterality, 30% bilaterality with BRC1-BRC2 mutations.
4. A patient with one-sided breast cancer infiltrating lobular carcinoma or medullar breast cancer is at increased risk of bilaterality.

5. A patient with one-sided breast cancer associated with DCIS and LCIS is at increased risk of bilaterality.

FINDINGS FROM MEDICAL LITERATURE

Frequency of bilaterality of breast cancer.

1. By mammography reported 6% in 112 breast cancer (EGAN).
2. By MRI reported 24% bilaterality in high-risk patients and 10% in non-high-risk patients (Lehman).
3. By surgery reported 22% bilaterality of breast cancer in reduction mammoplasty (Mascarel).
4. By random surgical biopsy of the opposite breast reported 11% breast cancer (Urban).
5. It is also reported in the literature that the risk of breast cancer in the opposite breast is 0.5 to 0.8 per year versus 0.1 per year in general female population.
6. *Autopsy findings:* This is the most accurate information about bilaterality of breast cancer. Nielsen et al. published findings in Cancer in 1986 of eighty-four autopsies of patient who died of breast cancer. In 68% primary cancer was found in the opposite breast; 33% was invasive and 35% was DCIS, also 16% metastasis from other organs, except in eight cases—the rest were not suspected clinically and found in autopsy. 71% had axillary lymph node metastasis. One of the most important finding was that the mean survival of patients with bilateral breast cancer was compatible with survival of patients who died of unilateral breast cancer. It is also reported in the literature by others that only in 7% of cases of bilaterality breast cancer prognostically were worse than unilateral breast cancer.

In 1997, in the screening mammography on the right breast of a forty-eight-year-old patient, a small 8 mm well-differentiated invasive cancer was found. No axillary lymph node metastasis, lumpectomy, and radiation were performed. Ten months later, the patient felt a mass in her left breast. Mammography one year later showed 6 cm comet-type cancerous mass. Surgery revealed undifferentiated invasive carcinoma, grade III, four lymph nodes involved with metastasis worse outcome than the first right-side breast cancer.

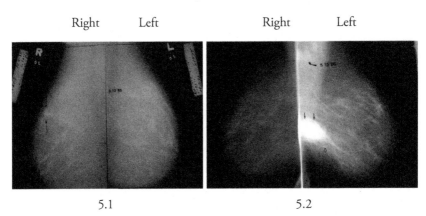

5.1

In 1985 small nodule of breast cancer between arrows

5.2

In 1986 less than 1 year a large cancer developed on the left side white color mass (arrows) with lymph node metastasis.

We learn from these findings that bilaterality of breast cancer is more common than reported in the literature:

1. Bilaterality of breast cancer occurs more in high-risk patients.
2. Patients with one-sided breast cancer are at high risk to develop breast cancer in the opposite breast in 68% of autopsies.
3. Patients with one-sided breast cancer are at high risk to develop cancer in other organs. This risk is 13%.
4. 68% of patients die with undetected bilateral breast cancer (discovered in autopsy).
5. As the patient ages, frequency of bilaterality increases.

6. Patients with one-sided breast cancer requesting bilateral mastectomy in 93% do not gain any survival benefits.
7. 7% of cancer of the opposite side is of worse prognosis. (One case is reported here.)
8. The most important finding is that survival of patients with bilateral breast cancer is almost equal to the survival of patients with one-sided breast cancer.
9. We learned that when we detect breast cancer in one breast by screening mammography, MRI of the breast should be performed; in the previous case we would have found left breast cancer sooner.

CHAPTER 6

RISK FACTORS IN BREAST CANCER

A large number of elements have been reported in the literature as a promoter of breast cancer. The ones that have a scientific basis are described in this book.

Gender, age, menopausal status, genetics, x-ray. Debatable risk factors are hormones and trauma.

Gender: The highest risk factor for breast cancer is to be a female. 99% of the time cancer develops in females and 1% in men.

Age: Risk for breast cancer parallels aging. For instance, at the age of forty, one case of cancer out of 225; at the age of sixty, one case in 24; and at the age of eighty-five, 13% one case in 8 (cumulative risk).

Menopausal status: Approximately two-thirds of newly diagnosed breast cancer are in patients of equal or more than fifty years old.

Genetic factor: All breast cancers are subsequent to genetic changes called mutation. Damaged genes before conception called germ-line mutation or hereditary breast cancer are transmitted to the offspring. This cancer usually develops before the age of menopause. Gene damage after conception causing cancer is called sporadic breast cancer. In hereditary breast cancer, damaged genes located in chromosome XIII and XVII, also called BRC1+ and BRC2+, increase the risk of breast cancer to 85% at the age of seventy. Ovarian cancer lifetime risk in normal female population is 2%. In mutated BRC1 the risk increases to 63% and with BRC2 to 16%.

In Ashkenazim ethnicity two protein mutations in BRC1 and one mutation in BRC2 have been reported, which raises the risk of breast cancer to 56% by the age of seventy. These mutations are carried in about 2.5% of female population. It should be mentioned that a very low percentage of female population have BRC1 and BRC2 mutations without family history of breast carcinoma. Females with BRC1+ and BRC2+ have a higher incidence of bilateral breast cancer and other organs—ovarian, colon, pancreas—and it is because damaged genes are present in all cells of the body. This is not in sporadic breast cancer.

X-RAY AS A HIGH-RISK FACTOR FOR BREAST CANCER

Solar rays contain a large spectrum of rays of different energies. Lower energy is found in ultraviolet and infrared, and high energy in x-rays and gamma rays. Infrared and ultraviolet with their low energy cannot penetrate deep into our bodies. They are absorbed superficially but can occasionally promote skin cancer. X-rays and gamma rays, mainly industrial type, have powerful energy and penetrate deep in our organs and can cause damage to our genes, thus promoting cancer. The most vulnerable organs to x-rays are breasts, ovaries, testicles, thyroid, skin, and blood cells. It has been reported scientifically that in the following conditions more cancer has been seen.

1. More breast cancer has been seen in workers of radium paintings (old fluorescent watches).
2. Higher incidences of breast cancer have been noted in airline hostesses. The higher the altitude, the higher the exposure to x-rays and gamma rays. This is why astronauts wear special protective suits.
3. With the atomic bomb explosion in Hiroshima and Nagasaki, ninety thousand people were exposed to radiation. It doubled the number of breast cancer after thirty

years in patients whose ages were younger than thirty years at the time of the explosion.
4. In a Dutch study published in *Journal American Medical Association*, in 551 women ages twenty-five to fifty who were treated for Hodgkin's lymphoma before the age of twenty-one with moderate dose of x-ray radiation at the age of forty-five, 20% of the patients developed breast cancer.
5. Radiation Oncology (June 2009) of Massachusetts General Hospital Harvard Medical School published thirty-nine cases of breast cancer sixteen years after radiotherapy for Hodgkin's lymphoma. Twenty-eight patients were at the age of twenty-five and forty-five when they were treated; 39% developed bilateral breast carcinoma.
6. In a group of patients treated for pneumothorax with frequent fluoroscopy in 1930 to 1950 or patients who had x-ray therapy for post-partum mastitis from 1940 to 1920 and patients with ankylosing spondylosis 1930 to 1950 treated with x-ray had developed more breast cancer after about twenty years of their treatment.
7. In December of 2008, in the *Journal of Clinical Oncology* comparing the risk of cancer in the opposite breast (contralateral) in women who were treated in 1986 with radiation after lumpectomy, it was found that (a) before the age forty-five, the women had 1.5-fold increased risk of cancer in the opposite breast and (b) younger women who had strong family history of breast cancer had 3.5-fold increased risk of breast cancer.
8. In randomized trials of European Organizations for Research and Treatment for Cancer (EORTC) in two groups their first report shows that the group who had lumpectomy and radiation therapy had developed three times more breast cancer in the opposite breast than the group that did not receive radiation therapy. X-ray radiation, which may stimulate breast cancer, is thought to be about 200 rads (2GY). In radiotherapy of breast cancer, at

least that amount of x-ray can be absorbed by contralateral breast.
9. Induced x-ray breast carcinoma in the same breast such as angiosarcoma has been reported ten to fifteen years after radiation therapy in conservative treatment.
10. In 2009 according to the national council on radiation protection and measurement, the American population is seven times more exposed to x-ray and gamma radiation than in 1980. Radiation per capita of American population rose from 15% to 48%. American population is only 4.6% of the world population, but 50% of all types of radiation for medical diagnosis and treatment is used in the USA. Alarming figure was that twenty-nine thousand cancers in 2007 were induced by CT scan.

Can screening mammography cause breast cancer?

It has never been shown and never can be shown the threshold of medical x-ray that can cause breast cancer. Patients having four sets of mammography, two for each side, get 1 rad of x-ray, which is far from 200 rads, which is theoretically admitted to be carcinogenic. Risk calculation up to now has been based on extrapolation from relatively high-dose x-ray exposure as mentioned before. The risk of breast cancer by screening mammography is low but certainly not zero. Theoretically, ten years of annual screening mammography can cause one case of breast cancer in ten thousand females.

We learn from these data that x-ray exposure can cause breast cancer. In order to reduce the risk we should avoid x-ray exposure as much as possible, including diagnostic x-ray or therapy by x-ray and airport x-ray checking, especially in young age and during pregnancy.

CHAPTER 7

DEBATABLE RISK FACTOR IN BREAST CANCER

1. Are hormones risk factors for breast cancer?

Two incriminated hormones are estrogen and progesterone secreted by the ovaries from young age to menopause. They participate in at least forty vital functions in the female body. Some mammals cannot survive without hormones. Chimpanzees that are genetically very close to humans die after menopause at forty-five to fifty years of age. Menopause for chimpanzees is a dead end, but for human females it is a new era, a long way to go and to cope with the sign of the lack of hormones. Not long ago average age longevity of females was fifty-five years. Nowadays it is eighty years. Signs of lack of hormone in pre-menopausal as well as post-menopausal females, such as hot flashes, osteoporosis, vascular trouble, headaches, irritability, moodiness and night sweats, loss of memory, signs of depression, insomnia, vaginal dryness, urogenital infection, bladder atonia, Alzheimer's, and lack of sex are common and are consequences of ovary retirement or ovarian surgery and the dryness of fountain of youth. Prior to 2002 physicians advocated hormone replacement therapy (HRT) in post-menopausal females with relatively good results. Physicians did not have any fear of causing breast cancer or cardiovascular complications. From 1995 to 2000 more than sixty-five papers published about post-menopausal hormone replacement in 80% of them showed overwhelming benefits and no increase of breast cancer. In 2002, *Women's Health Initiative* (WHI) changed the whole history. The research was done by correspondence over two groups of post-menopausal female aging fifty to seventy-nine years. A group of 8,506 females were given daily 0.65 mg of estrogen and 2.5 mg of progesterone. The other group of 8,102 females were given no hormones (placebo). The research was planned for eight years, but it stopped abruptly in 5.2 years because in their view an excess of breast cancer was found in the group taking hormones. The result was published as follows:

Risks of hormones seen in the group of women taking hormones

- 38 cases of breast cancer in 10,000 per year in the group taking hormones versus 30 cases of breast cancer in 10,000 per year in the group not taking hormones; relative risk reported to be 1.36
- Coronary heart disease: 7 more per 10,000 per year
- Strokes: 8 more per 10,000 per year when compared with the placebo

Benefits of hormones seen in the group of women taking hormones

- Reduction of colorectal cancer: 6 less per 10,000
- Reduction of hip fracture: 5 less per 10,000
- The most important finding: No change in breast cancer survival in either groups (taking or not taking hormones)

This minimal excess of breast cancer in the group taking hormones was magnified to such a level by mass media that overnight all over the world, millions of females stopped taking their hormones. However, three important findings on the benefit of hormone in reduction of osteoporosis and, particularly, a worse type of cancer—colorectal cancer—and equal survival in both groups were not blown up or trumpeted and remained silent by mass media. If we study carefully this trial like many other trials, weak points can be noticed: flaws inherent to any large medical trials performed by numerous institutions, in this case in forty sites. In this study, 42% stopped taking hormones and 38% from the placebo took hormones, noncompliances; pollution seen also in this trial may affect noticeably the results. Excess of breast cancer, 8 more per 10,000, is not statistically sound and powerful for scientific statisticians who state, "Forget it if it is less than three times."

Authors of WHI research mention excess of breast cancer <u>almost reached nominal statistical significance</u>. As Dr. Blooming, a master of the American College of Physicians and professor of medicine at USC, in his publication about the WHI findings, said, "When you say 'almost' it means it did not reach statistical significance." A propos of reported coronary heart disease, seven more per ten thousand and stroke eight more per ten thousand, it was not specified what the ages were of those patients when they started to take hormones. We know that if hormones are taken long after menopause (sixty-five to seventy), they increase the risk of thromboemboli and vascular sickness.

Authors of the research reported no increase in early stage of breast cancer (DCIS). If hormones really increased breast cancer, the first thing that we should have seen would have been the increase of DCIS progenitors of invasive cancer.

Authors of the research reported also no difference on mammographic findings in both groups. Again, if hormone causes breast cancer, the first thing that we should have seen is the increase of detection of cancer by mammography. This did not happen either. After the publication of the research, a storm of critics unleashed. Paul Brunner, professor of obstetrics and gynecology at Obstetrics and Gynecology at USC, called Women's Health Initiative a national tragedy.

Dr. Blooming reported strong convincing documents invalidating the WHI finding in breast cancer that did not provoke any publicity. In 2003 the WHI published a follow-up of the incidence of breast cancer which was reported lower, 1.24 less than in 2002, which was 1.36. In 2005 and in 2011, WHI updated their research showing the following on estrogen-alone trial:

- After stopping estrogen among post-menopausal women who had prior hysterectomy, at the end of 10.7 years of total follow-up, there was significant reduced risk of breast cancer.
- Women who began estrogen therapy while in their fifties had reduced risk of heart attacks, death, and less colorectal cancer.
- Women who started estrogen therapy in their seventies had an increased risk of overall illness and death and an increased risk of colorectal cancer.
- Regarding the use of estrogen and progesterone in patients with signs of lack of hormone short-term, low-dose can be given, and in surgical menopausal, high dose is appropriate.
- For long-term use of estrogen and progesterone in asymptomatic females, balance of risks and benefits should be evaluated, starting with low dose for shortest periods of time.

CONTROVERSIES OF HORMONES IN BREAST CANCER

In 1896, Beatson, MD, published the remission of metastasis of breast cancer after removal of the ovaries. Since that time, it was thought that the excess of ovarian hormone, particularly estrogen, can cause breast cancer. It is shown experimentally in laboratory animals that estrogen can provoke and promote breast cancer. In humans, it is also shown that estrogen can greatly accelerate the growth of estrogen receptor positive DCIS in xenograft, whereas the growth in ER receptor negative implant was ineffective. It is reported also that the risk of breast cancer increases when estrogen is used in combination with progesterone; progesterone is reported to be the culprit.

Questions without answers:

If excess of hormones can cause breast cancer, why is breast cancer three times more in post-menopausal women who have much less ovarian hormones than premenopausal women?

Contraceptive pills contain more estrogen and progesterone taken by patients in whom less breast cancer develops than the nonuser. Study in women who had hysterectomy and using estrogen alone showed no increase in breast cancer risk.

During pregnancy or breast-feeding, the highest amount of hormones circulates in the female body. No more breast cancer is seen in those situations. Pregnancy after breast cancer treatment is not detrimental to the patient's survival.

For more than half a century, hormone, estrogen, progesterone, and testosterone have been given to patients to stop the progression of breast cancer metastasis of stage IV after exhaustion of all other medications. Still, today, they are the most efficient treatment for metastasis of breast cancer with long remission, but they are less used today because of side effects.

Hormone estrogen has been given to patients who have been treated for breast cancer because of the development of the intolerable sign of lack of hormones for intense hot flashes; it has not affected the survival of the patients when compared with a nonuser who had been treated for breast cancer. Why ninety percent of men's breast cancer is estrogen-receptors positive despite of their lesser estrogen.

COMPARISON OF BREAST CANCER RISK OF HORMONE WITH OTHER RISK FACTORS AS REPORTED IN THE LITERATURE

Hormones: 1.24	Diabetes: 2.3
Alcohol: 1.26	Left-handed: 2.41
French fries: 1.27	Family history of breast cancer: 2.76
Grapefruit: 1.30	Past breast biopsies: 2.9
Night shift: 1.51, 1.70	Electric blanket: 4.9
Breast fibroadenoma: 1.7	Vitamin D deficiency: 5.83
Flight attendants: 1.87	Smoking: 7

| Antibiotics: 2.07 | BRC1 and BRC2 positive: 7 |

This means that in order to reduce breast cancer risks, not only hormones which have the least risk to promote breast cancer should be eliminated, but grapefruit, antibiotics, female flight attendant jobs, electric blankets should also be avoided.

The role of hormones in causing breast cancer in humans is not clear.

Even if hormones cause breast cancer, the risk is minimal, doubtedly overrides the benefits. Unfortunately, before knowing the exact role of hormones and its risk for breast cancer, precipitously we deprived irrationally millions of females who badly needed hormones, suffering from side effects and disease caused by the lack of hormones. Fortunately after the passage of time, researchers recognized the role of hormones in the well-being of females, and the risk of breast cancer is not as alarming as it was thought, and they recommended hormones in certain circumstances.

Conclusion: Hormones are normal and indispensable food for our body cells. The role of hormones in causing breast cancer in humans is not proven, but its contribution to the growth of cancer has been shown not for all breast cancer but only in breast cancer with estrogen receptor positive. Therefore, it is a promoter and not and instigator. We should make a distinction between causation and promotion.

2. ELECTRIC LIGHT RISK FACTOR IN BREAST CANCER

MORE SCIENTIFC WORK HAS BEEN DONE FOR NIGHT-SHIFT WORKERS

FINDINGS IN NIGHT-SHIFT WORKERS

Our cells, like all living creatures and plants, have a circadian system, which is regulated by laws of nature established after rotation of our planet, forming day and night. There are functions in the cells that are performed uniquely in daylight and others in the dark of the night; this constant revolving function is called circadian rhythmicity, which is directed by a gene called clock gene. In the past it has been observed and reported that breast cancer is less common in blind women and also more common in women working in the night shift than the day shift. One of the hallmarks of civilization is the increased use of electricity to light the night, unnatural exposure of human to light, violating the laws of nature, disrupting the circadian rhythmicity of the cell, which may run us into problems. A hormone called melatonin is secreted in the dark (night) by the pineal gland in the brain. Now it is proven that melatonin has two main functions; one is causing sleeping, the other suppressing breast cancer formation. In the night shift, electric lighting rich in blue wavelength is more effective than yellow in disrupting circadian rhythmicity, and by disturbing clock gene, which control the cell's cycle, it may result in DNA mutation and formation of cancer. Acid lineolic in the breast is a promoting factor of breast cancer; melatonin in the breast cells is a suppressor factor of acid lineolic. It has been shown that light exposure at night markedly increases the growth of human breast cancer grafted in rat (xenograft). Blask et al. demonstrated that perfusion of human breast cancer xenograft in nude rats by blood taken from young women during the day, **during the night (dark)**, and during night, but women exposed to the light, only blood taken **during the night (dark)**, containing high degree of melatonin, strongly inhibited the growth of xenograft cancer. It is reported that bright light from bedside lamp, TV, computer screen, and tablets suppresses melatonin in all sighted persons, disturbs the timing of circadian rhythm, and elevates alertness and makes it harder to fall asleep. Exposure to the blue light at night causing circadian disruption is particularly important for children, also in pregnant women, which may affect their fetuses. It is also reported that in breast cancer, patients exposed to night light exhibit increased resistance to respond to the effect of chemo therapy and anti-hormone therapy.

Analogy exists between breast cancer in women and prostate cancer in men. Researchers have found that when men working at night shift, their hormone PSA (prostatic specific antigen), normally 4 ng/

ml, increases to more than 10 ng/ml. This is an elevated risk factor for developing prostatic cancer.

In conclusion, night is for sleeping. Avoid as much as possible exposing ourselves to the bright light, particularly blue-enriched compact fluorescent lightbulb.

3. TRAUMA RISK FACTOR OF BREAST CANCER

Classically, trauma is not reported in medical literature as a risk factor, but we have documents that it can cause breast cancer. We report it here as a risk factor and present several cases. If we look back to the old medical literature in the early seventeenth century, we will find that trauma to the breast causing breast cancer has been reported, incriminating blow to the breast, tight clothes, and rough handling as major factors. Even in 1912, Dr. Handley advised prophylactic course of x-ray after trauma to the breast in order to prevent development of cancer. In recent literature, 9% to 26% of women attributed their breast cancer to the trauma. However, Dr. Haagensen, world-renowned American surgeon, in his textbook, doubted that trauma can cause breast cancer. Why this controversy? In the past, physicians did not have opportunities of documentation as we have nowadays by mammography, ultrasonography, and MRI. If a patient develops a mass later at the site of the trauma, screening mammography done before trauma showed no abnormality; now mammography shows an abnormal image corresponding to the mass. It can be either a cancer or a fat necrosis (benign). Abnormal images can be specific: round eggshell calcified mass consisting of fat necrosis. If the image is not specific, round or irregular speculated mass or appearance of group of microcalcifications are highly suspicious for malignancy, and core needle biopsy should be performed. It should be said that fat necrosis sometimes mimics breast cancer clinically, mammographically and cytologically done by fine needle aspiration; we should not trust the report of the pathologist, and core needle biopsy should be performed. Breast cancer incidence after breast trauma is much higher than we think. Patients forget often their trauma, and the physician never asks them.

Our observations:

1. A forty-eight-year-old patient in 1994 had a screening mammography and a normal physical examination with us. Eight months later, patient had car accident, causing extensive seat belt injury to the right upper outer quadrant of the breast, causing bruises and bleeding. The wound healed in two months. Six months after the trauma, the patient felt hardening at the site of injury. She saw a doctor who told her that is common after trauma. The patient came in 1996 from another state to see us. On physical examination, a palpable mass was felt in the right upper outer quadrant as well as axillary lymph nodes. Mammography demonstrated an irregular mass in the right upper outer quadrant with multiple dense axillary lymph nodes. Surgery confirmed 2.5 cm invasive ductal carcinoma with four lymph node metastasis. The patient received conservative treatment and radiation and chemotherapy, and she was seen in 2007, alive but with distant metastasis.

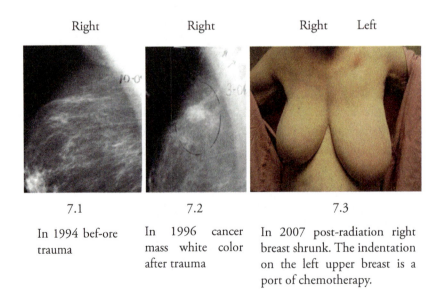

7.1 In 1994 before trauma

7.2 In 1996 cancer mass white color after trauma

7.3 In 2007 post-radiation right breast shrunk. The indentation on the left upper breast is a port of chemotherapy.

2. A seventy-two-year-old healthy woman, a physician, had a hard elbow hit to the middle of her right breast. The patient felt a sharp pain followed by swelling. After a while, the swelling regressed. One and a half years after the trauma, the patient noted and felt a mass exactly at the same point of the previous hit. As a physician, she thought that would be a residual hematoma or a benign condition. She neglected any consultation because of no pain, fever, or discomfort until she noticed the mass ulcerated to the skin. We saw the patient two years and three months after the trauma. Mammography showed 5 cm irregular mass with numerous axillary lymph node densities. Mastectomy demonstrated invasive ductal carcinoma with eight axillary lymph node metastasis.

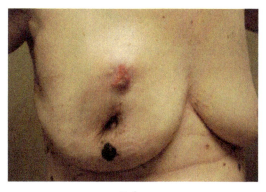 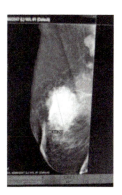

7.4

Upper round red spot is the outbreak of cancer to the skin. In the middle oval dark is nipple retracted; lower round dark is a mole.

7.5

Lateral right side mammography large white mass is breast cancer with multiple lymph node metastasis in the axilla.

3. On December 1990, a healthy fifty-three-year-old woman had a car crash accident causing bruises on her left breast and shoulder; she was seen because of pain on her breast. Mammography showed nonspecific lesion; ultrasound showed no mass. Patient was requested to be seen in six months but came back one and a half year later with palpable mass on the left outer side of the left breast. Mammography showed large irregular mass density on the same place of the previous trauma. Surgery showed 4 cm invasive ductal carcinoma (fig. 7.6 and 7.7); thirty-six out of forty axillary lymph nodes were involved with metastasis (fig. 7.10).

Photography	Mammography	Left Photography	Mammography Left
7.6	7.7	7.8	7.9
in 1990 car crash bruise on the left breast	1.5 year later cancer white mass on the left upper outer quadrant	In 1994 left breast seat belt injury	In 1996 cancer was diagnosed at the site of previous injury white mass

4. Another fifty-eight-year-old patient in 1994 (fig. 7.8 and 7.9); left breast seat belt injury, two years later breast cancer (fig. 7.11).
5. A healthy fifty-three-year-old woman was kicked eight months earlier by her horse to the right breast. The patient had bruises, bleeding, and swelling, which all regressed in a few weeks. But the patient felt constant dull pain. She came for a screening mammography, which showed more density in the middle of the right breast with clustered microcalcifications. At first we thought of fat necrosis.

Core needle biopsy revealed ductal carcinoma in situ and invasive cancer.

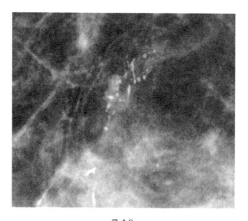

7.10

Magnification of right side mammography shows very well microcalcifications, small white particles seen in breast cancer.

6. A forty-year-old patient was seen in June 1996 because of small soft nodule at the right twelve o'clock position which appeared after a trauma occurred two months earlier. The patient ran into a wardrobe rock in the garment department. Mammography, ultrasonography, and fine needle aspiration were negative. Patient was seen six months later. The nodule was slightly larger. Ultrasonography showed benign type of image. Fine needle aspiration was done. Pathology reported typical fat necrosis. Patient was requested to be seen six months later. At this time, the nodule was larger in size. Mammography showed nonspecific density. Ultrasonography again showed larger benign type of image. Core needle biopsy showed ductal invasive carcinoma. Surgery revealed 3 cm cancer with four lymph node positive.

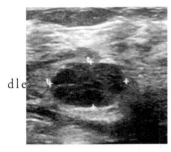

Breast ultrasonography of patient

Dark oval-shaped image looks like a benign lesion, but it is a cancer. Clinical examination, mammography, ultrasonography, and fine needle aspiration all were misleading. Only core needle biopsy unveiled the culprit cancer.

7.11. Image of solid mass of cancer, well-defined borders mimicking benign lesion (fibroadenoma or fat necrosis)

For comparison:

Image of cyst, black oval shape with regular borders

Irregular black image consistent with breast cancer

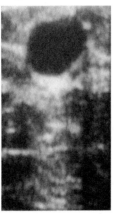

7.12

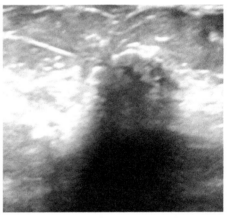

7.13

We learn from these observations the following:

- Trauma to the breast causes large area of breast tissue laceration probably causing breast cancer development.
- Cancer can be developed after direct breast trauma (e.g., blow to the breast, seat belt injury from car crash) and appears at the same area no more than two years later.
- Cancers appearing after trauma are fast-growing and highly lymphogenic.

- After trauma, two types of tumor may appear in the breast. One is fat necrosis (benign) and the other breast cancer (malignant).
- Sometimes, fat necrosis mimics all signs of breast cancer.
- Any developing mass after breast trauma should have core needle biopsy, unless typical sign of calcified mass is seen on mammography consistent with fat necrosis. We should not trust fine needle aspiration cytology (patient no. 6).
- After trauma, patient should be examined clinically and by ultrasonography every six months as well as annual mammography for the first two years.
- Prevention: To avoid breast trauma, if possible, the most troubling item is seat belt with sharp edges that not only in car crashes injures the breast but may also cut the vessels of the neck and throat. For that we need a law for manufacturing a safe and soft-edged seat belts.

4. BRASSIERE SYNDROME AND RELATION TO BREAST CANCER REPORTED IN THE LITERATURE

In Europe and the USA, brassiere syndrome and its connection with breast cancer have been previously published. In 1991, a study from Harvard published in the European *Journal of Cancer* stated that bra-free women had half the incidence of breast cancer than those wearing a bra. A study in England showed that the longer a woman wears a bra, the more likely she is to have breast cancer. In 1995, a book called *Dressed to Kill* by Cindy Ross Singer and Soma Grismajer, anthropologist, published and claimed that women who wore a tighter-fitting bra all day every day had a much higher risk of developing breast cancer than those who went au natural. Authors thought that cancer was caused by restriction of lymph flow in the breast. However, their assumption was not documented. There is no doubt that the compression of any organ can cause circulatory disturbances, but there is no proof that can provoke the genesis of cancer. In fact, a million of females have gotten implants and breast augmentations, which can cause serious compression, periprosthetic reaction, and fibrosis, causing circulatory disturbances, but no more cancer is seen in these females than those of the general population.

UNTOLD RISK FACTOR

UNDERWIRE BRASSIERE SYNDROME AND ITS RELATION TO BREAST CANCER (NOT REPORTED IN THE LITERATURE)

We report more specific syndrome called "underwire brassiere syndrome, author's observations."

In this book we report a large number of underwire brassiere syndrome and the relation with breast cancer. Development of cancer by chronic rubbing and friction of the skin with hard material (environmental carcinoma) is not a new finding. First, a British surgeon, Dr. Pott, documented cancer in some working professions such as in chimney boys (fireplace sweeper boys), ascending and descending naked body, scrapping against the chimney's wall covered with tar and soot. In the long run, some of them developed a fatal cancer of the scrotum. In French literature, development of skin cancer in the back of the chimney sweepers has been reported as well. We have observed and have proofs that brassieres with hard band such as underwire, by constant pressure, rubbing in semicircular manner the side and underside of the breast after years, in certain females, can cause breast cancer. But before that happens, there are numerous warning signs (underwire syndrome). The signs are worse if the brassiere is worn for twenty-four hours. These signs are the following:

1. Pain. Tight brassiere can cause pain particularly when the breasts are not of equal sizes. The pain is always in the larger side.
2. Skin lesion depends on the texture of the skin and the duration of wearing underwire brassiere. In the beginning, a faint redness may develop. Later, continuous friction wears off the top layer of the skin leading to intense red-

ness, abrasion, and fissure with exzematoid alteration. In some other patients, after long standing, combination of pimples, acne, and warts are seen. In the worse scenario, fissures appear underneath the breast, sometimes with bacterial dermatitis and malodorous fungal infection (candidiasis). In dark skin, thickening, hyperpigmentation, and likenification can develop. In young people, only skin thickening can be seen. Breast cancer that we have seen developed in semicircular line around the breast where the underwire presses hard particularly underneath the breast. That is where we discover bilateral breast cancer, and for us that was the most convincing proof that underwire brassiere can provoke breast cancer.

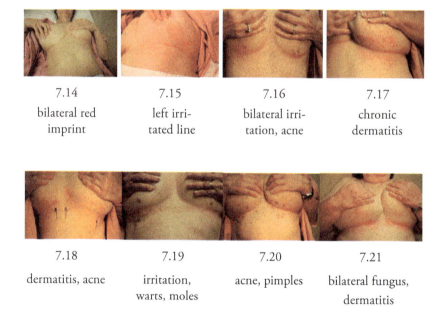

7.14 bilateral red imprint

7.15 left irritated line

7.16 bilateral irritation, acne

7.17 chronic dermatitis

7.18 dermatitis, acne

7.19 irritation, warts, moles

7.20 acne, pimples

7.21 bilateral fungus, dermatitis

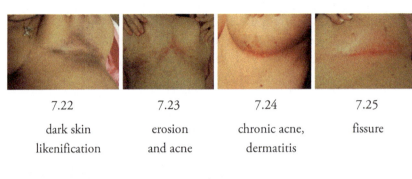

7.22	7.23	7.24	7.25
dark skin likenification	erosion and acne	chronic acne, dermatitis	fissure

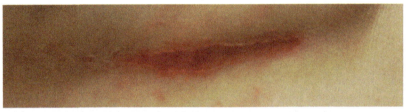

Only by magnification can we realize the extent of the damage of the underwire brassiere.

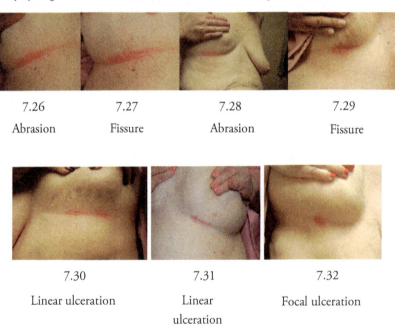

7.26	7.27	7.28	7.29
Abrasion	Fissure	Abrasion	Fissure

7.30	7.31	7.32
Linear ulceration	Linear ulceration	Focal ulceration

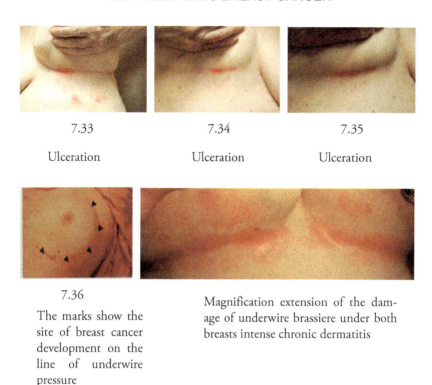

7.33 Ulceration

7.34 Ulceration

7.35 Ulceration

7.36
The marks show the site of breast cancer development on the line of underwire pressure

Magnification extension of the damage of underwire brassiere under both breasts intense chronic dermatitis

3. Frequency of breast cancer: In American women, 25% to 30% of cancer develops in semicircular line close to the chest wall corresponding to the site of the underwire pressure. It is interesting to know that in North America and Europe breast cancer develops in 125 per 100,000 female per years. In Japan it is 28 per 100,000, and in China 20 per 100,000. However, when the Japanese or Chinese migrate to the USA, their offspring born in America develop the same number of breast cancer as those native in America. Tight underwire brassieres have been worn for centuries in America and in Europe, which can contribute to the development of more cancer. Recently, chronic inflammation of tissue in any organ has been reported as a high risk for the genesis of cancer. Trauma to the breast can cause microinjuries, lacerations, and chronic inflammation inside the breast tissue, which can contribute to the genesis of breast cancer.

The first observation:

1. A fifty-three-year-old woman in 1991 had a screening mammography with us, and no abnormality was seen. But on physical examination, intense local redness, small fissure, and skin thickening were found underneath both breasts, interpreted as a simple skin sweating and irritation. We did not know that this was caused by her underwire brassiere. We requested a one-year follow-up. In 1992, the screening mammography showed no abnormality, and the physical examination showed larger fissure with much harder skin and redness underneath both breasts. Fine needle aspiration cytology showed fat necrosis. Only as a measure of precaution, because of the worsening of clinical findings, surgical biopsy was performed in both suspicious areas and astonishingly revealed bilateral invasive breast cancer. If we had not seen bilateral cancer at six o'clock symmetrically after long-wear (thirty years) underwire bra, we could have never imagined that an underwire bra could cause breast cancer. Following this, we were looking for such events, and we found numerous cases of unilateral breast cancer in semicircular line or underneath the breast after twenty-five- to thirty-year wear of underwire bra.

Following are cancers detected in different patients, different ages wearing underwire bra more than twenty years shown here with their corresponding mammography.

FIGHT NEW WAYS BREAST CANCER

1992 Right Left   Right 1996   Right Left

7.37 Photo shows bilateral 6 o'clock breast cancer

7.38 Mammography after radiation bilateral scars small white images close to the chest wall

7.39 6 o'clock breast cancer on the line of the underwire pressure

7.40 Mammography after radiation Right breast shrink, scar formation close to chest wall

1998 Right Left   2000   Right Left

7.41 6 o'clock right breast cancer

7.42 Scar density 6 o'clock after radiation

7.43 6 o'clock left breast cancer

7.44 After radiation left breast shrunk, calcified scar at 6 o'clock

Left 2000   Right Left   Right 2000   Right 2002

7.45 5 o'clock left breast cancer

7.46 After radiation left breast small scar white image close to the chest wall

7.47 Cancer at 8 o'clock on the line of pressure

7.48 Cancer at 7 o'clock at the pressure line

We learn from these observations the following:

1. Any hard band, particularly underwire brassiere, might provoke in the long term invasive breast cancer by laceration and chronic inflammation of breast tissue. More breast cancer is seen in the Western countries probably because of more usage of underwire bra.
2. Majority of cancer develop in semicircular line, particularly underneath the breasts where more compression and rubbing are exercised (fig. 7.36).
3. Because of the closeness and adhesions of cancer to the chest wall underneath the breast, cancer cannot be projected on mammography; if the radiologist does not examine the patient, this can easily be missed.
4. Often, before the formation of cancer, different types of skin lesions can be seen, mainly underneath the breasts. If the breasts are not lifted up, even a large breast lesion can be overlooked. In many occasions, the patient herself was not aware of ulceration. Sometimes the patient would be treated for itching and for a long time with Cortisone without results.
5. A large number of chronic pain of the breasts are due to the tight brassiere with more pain on the larger side (more compression).
6. Fine needle aspiration may report fat necrosis (benign lesion); we should not trust that diagnosis, and core needle or open surgical biopsy should be performed in suspicious lesion. Treatment and prevention are simple, not using any tight or hard underband brassiere.

CHAPTER 8

METHODS OF BREAST CANCER DETECTION

1. Physical examination
2. Film, digital mammography, and tomosynthesis
3. MRI, spectrography MRI
4. Ultrasonography, hand-held or automatic; elastography
5. Ductography
6. Nuclear medicine, PEM (positron emission mammography), PET scan (positron emission tomography)
7. SPEM (single photon emission mammography)

METHODS OF BREAST CANCER DIAGNOSIS

1. Fine needle aspiration cytology
2. Core needle biopsy without or with mammography (stereotactic) or under the control of ultrasonography, or MRI
3. Punch biopsy of the skin
4. Open surgical biopsy

Diagnosis of breast cancer is made by microscopy of tissue or by genetics of cells.

PHYSICAL EXAMINATION OF THE BREAST (NEGLECTED ART)

Physical examination of the breast is the oldest way to find breast cancer.

Clinical signs of breast cancer:

There are signs caused by cancer that can be seen, can be felt, and can be sensed by the patient. In the beginning of the breast cancer development, there is no sign. In later stages, it is manifested by different signs such as breast discomfort, vague pain (intermittent or constant), unilateral nipple bloody discharge, nipple erosion, nipple eczema, nipple inversion, nipple retraction, localized skin dimpling, coin-size retracted chronic ulceration, bleeding, infected, ulcerated breast mass, large number of breast cancer manifested by indolent nodule found from lentil-size mobile under the skin to a firm, fixed orange-size mass or enlarging axillary lymph node due to metastasis with or without detectable lesion on mammography. Sometimes, breast cancer causes asymmetry of the breast. One side becomes smaller due to the entire retraction of the breast structure; other times, enlarging breast due to diffuse edematous cancer or inflammation with local or general discoloration and redness of the entire breast, called inflammatory breast cancer.

Inflammatory breast cancer is 1% of the total cancer and can be seen at any age during pregnancy or breast-feeding, usually on one side, exceptionally both sides (breast acute lymphoma). The breast becomes painful and gradually swells, the nipple retracts, the skin gets thicker and resembles an orange peel or peau d'orange, and the axillary lymph nodes enlarge. In this stage, the differentiation between inflammatory breast cancer and infection of the breast, called mastitis, is difficult. If a two-week course of antibiotics does not cause regression of the symptoms, punch biopsy of the skin will make the diagnosis possible. Any female noticing these signs should be seen by a physician.

DETECTING CANCER BY MAMMOGRAPHY: WHAT IS MAMMOGRAPHY?

Mammography is imaging of the breast structure, obtained by an x-ray machine. More than half a century it was known that breast cancer could be detected by mammography sooner than physical examination of the breast. In order to know whether this earlier diagnosis has any impact on survival, the first randomized trial was performed in the USA in 1960 by Health Insurance Plan of New York (called HIP), divided 62,000 females aged forty to seventy-four into two groups. The first group received annual physical examination and mammography for four years, and the second group nothing until the patient found an abnormality in her breast (placebo). The results after eight years and eighteen years showed 23% reduction of mortality in the group who had physical examination and mammography despite the fact that only 19% of breast cancer was found by mammography; the rest was found by physical examination and mammography. It showed that patients with the findings of cancer by annual physical examination and mammography had better survival than when the patient found the breast cancer herself. This test shows no survival benefits for patients forty to forty-nine years of age. Later, seven similar randomized trials were performed in Europe and in Canada. Total of eight randomizations, in six, reduction of 20% to 25% of mortality was reported, except one in Canadian and one in Sweden which showed no mortality reduction. This generated controversy and eternal debate for mammography, whether it is useful or not in forty- to forty-nine-year-old females. Despite this, the Cancer Society of American College of Radiologists and Gynecological Society advocated annual screening mammography after the age of forty; the rest of the world more or less followed the American Guideline Policy.

TECHNIQUE OF MAMMOGRAPHY

Two pictures are taken by x-ray from each breast in two directions for a total of four pictures. If a patient has implants, we have to displace the implant and take additional pictures because the implant hides breast tissue partially, thus resulting in a total of eight pictures. These are taken by trained and certified x-ray technologists. Their role is of paramount importance, not known by the public nor appraised by medical communities. What does mammography show us? Mammography shows the anatomy of the breast, its density, and normal or abnormal change of its structure. By abnormal changes we suspect cancer and lead to biopsy of the abnormality.

DENSITY OF THE BREAST: WHAT IS DENSE BREAST ON MAMMOGRAPHY?

If the breasts contain too many milk glands, more connective tissues, and more amorphous substance called collagen, the x-ray picture of the breast structure is white, called dense breast, seen in large majority in premenopausal females. When fat is predominant in the breast tissue, the picture of the breast is dark gray seen in large majority of post-menopausal females. There is a large spectrum of different tonalities of different densities and structures between those two extreme tonalities.

In dense breast the picture (fig. 8.2) is white because of superimposed compacted breast tissue. X-ray has difficulty to pass through and is largely absorbed by breast tissue. Contrarily, in predominant fatty breast (fig. 8.1), x-rays pass easily through the tissue and less x-ray is absorbed in the breast. Therefore, in small fatty breasts, the least amount of x-ray is absorbed by breast tissue, but much more x-ray is absorbed in the dense breasts, large breasts, breasts during pregnancy, during lactation, premenstrual, or breasts with implants. Dense breasts are reported to be in higher risk for breast cancer; it is certainly in higher risk of missing breast cancer because high density of breast tissue fogs image of cancer.

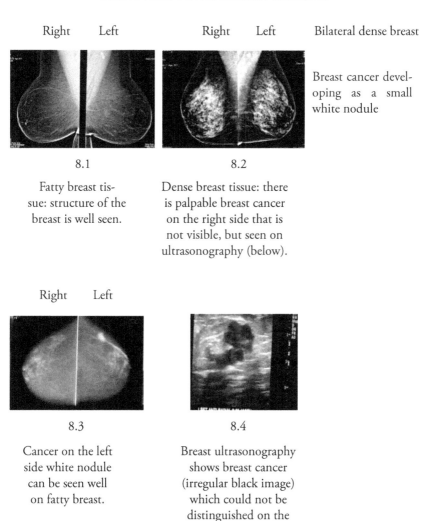

8.1 Fatty breast tissue: structure of the breast is well seen.

8.2 Dense breast tissue: there is palpable breast cancer on the right side that is not visible, but seen on ultrasonography (below).

8.3 Cancer on the left side white nodule can be seen well on fatty breast.

8.4 Breast ultrasonography shows breast cancer (irregular black image) which could not be distinguished on the above mammography.

INTERPRETATION OF MAMMOGRAPHY

Neither physician nor by far the public is aware of the difficulty of interpretation of mammography; it is the most difficult and most challenging task in all organ imaging in medical radiology, because the anatomy of the breast is composed of different structures, different shapes, and different consistency. Even in one individual, two breasts are different. The breast structure is not like other organs such as brain, heart, kidneys, liver, bones, etc., with steady structure in form and shape. We are looking at microchange in the structure of the breast whereas in other organs we are dealing with macrochange of anatomical structures. Each breast has a different structure. In fact, if there are three and a half billion females in the world, there are seven billion different structures and shapes of the breasts. It is similar to a fingerprint. In addition, breast anatomy changes accordion-like with different factors, with different amount of compression, different angle of projection, different time of the mammography. Breast structure changes with menstrual cycle, loss or gain of weight, pregnancy, breast-feeding, kidney or heart or vascular disease, drugs, medication, hormones, biopsy, surgery, reduction, augmentation, post-trauma, post-radiation, and benign and malignant lesions. Radiologist should be familiar with all aspects of the breast changes. Seventy percent of these changes mimic cancer, leading to biopsy of noncancerous lesions. Often we hear a patient telling us that mammography did not show her breast cancer. It is not the mammography that shows the breast cancer; it is the radiologist that should find invisible breast cancer in searching it in cloudy structures of the breasts (finding a needle in a haystack). When cancer is advanced, more or less has the same shape on mammography, mass with regular or irregular speculated borders, clustered microcalcifications, these can easily be seen even by nonmedical personnel. The difficulty arises in detection of early stage of breast cancer development. None of them look alike because the basic structure of the breast is different in each case (reported in author's book in 1996). A radiologist who has not seen thousands of breast cancer in early stage of development will have to face the reality; he or she will overlook breast cancer, which is happening unfortunately often. If we look to the published data even by prestigious university centers (IKEDA), they show that cancer detected today on mammography in 80% images of cancer but subtle were present on previous annual mammography undetected and reported normal. Author's book published in 1996 was based on studying 502 missed breast cancer on mammography; retrospective study of all previous screening mammography showed and taught us how a minuscule insignificant, uncharacteristic image of the breast density evolves and turns to a characteristic image of invasive cancer, image by which with long delay now we make diagnosis of breast cancer. It is extremely difficult to detect breast cancer on uncharacteristic presentations. In the past decade, all efforts have been done to remedy this shortcoming by creating in some universities breast imaging fellowship for one year, or Bi-Rad classification, legislation, computer aids, federal laws, a stringent measure for practicing mammography; they have all had a good result, but nothing can replace experience. Reading at least 10,000 mammographies a year for twenty years and having constant auto-audits of the result of biopsies are part of the solution. In our opinion, training, learning, and interpreting mammography is a lifetime experience.

MISSING OF BREAST CANCER BY SCREENING MAMMOGRAPHY

In my experience, physical examination by the radiologist correlating with mammography may be life-saving. However, it is not routinely done with screening mammography. We would have missed cancer in the following cases if we did not examine the patient:

1. Mammography cannot project the entire breast anatomy. Thus there are areas that are missing on mammography inherent to the anatomy of the breast tissue, particularly in the inner and lower sides of the breast. In these areas, cancer can be palpable and the patient unaware of it. If physical examination is not performed, cancer can be missed, and the result of mammography can be reported normal.
2. Cancer can develop in the area that can be projected on mammography, but because of malposition or inappropriate technique, those areas are not seen on mammography. Cancer in this area can be palpable. If physical examination is not performed, it can be missed, and the result of mammography can be reported normal.
3. There is about 20% of palpable breast cancer that causes no change on the structure of the breast, even with the

best mammography. If physical examination is not done, cancer can be missed, and the result of mammography can be reported normal.

4. Certain cancers invisible on mammography manifest first by palpable axillary lymph node metastasis. If physical examination is not done, cancer can be missed. If the radiologist examines the breast and finds a hard palpable mass in the axillary region, fine needle aspiration would demonstrate the presence of abnormal cells, then other test such as MRI or ultrasound of the breast might reveal the presence of invisible carcinoma on mammography. The report of mammography in this case can be normal.

5. Certain breast cancer manifests by nipple discharge, serous, clear, bloody without any other sign of breast cancer. Sometimes, the patient is unaware or paying no attention to it, forgets to mention it. If the patient is not examined, the radiologist cannot suggest other types of examination such as ductography, and cancer can be missed; the result of the screening mammography can be reported normal.

In all these cases the referring physician who relies on the report of the radiologist can be misled with undesirable consequences.

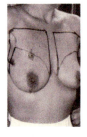
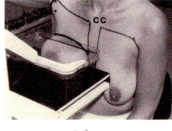
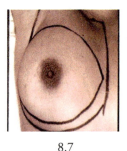

8.5	8.6	8.7
Breast tissue goes up to the clavicles: 2 black marks of cancer could not be projected on mammography.	Breast under compression: upper part of the breast tissue cannot be projected on mammography.	Double-lined area breast tissue cannot be well projected on mammography.

6. Breast cancer also can be missed on mammography because of subtle image of cancer. This is the most common elements of missing breast cancer but screening mammography reported normal. About 65% of breast cancer cannot be detected on mammography, but a larger number of them can be detected by MRI, but all of them can be found on microscopic mastectomy. This is the limitation of sensitivity of mammography. However, the future of screening belongs to three-dimensional imaging called tomosynthesis. On screening mammography, all structures of breasts are superimposed; in tomosynthesis by archway movement of x-ray tube, each layer of the breast tissue is imaged, and a lesion can be detected better. The only disadvantage is that it is costly and more x-ray is absorbed by the patient.

THE IMPORTANCE OF PRESENCE, SUPERVISION, AND PHYSICAL EXAMINATION BY RADIOLOGIST IN BREAST DISEASE

Missing slow-growing breast cancer may not affect survival, but missing fast-growing one may delay the treatment and have a great impact on the outcome of the patient. Missing breast cancer on screening mammography is the best trap for lawsuits, which may be devastating and career-ruining for radiologists and eventually for referring physicians. Lawsuits for missing breast cancer by radiologists are on the top of the list in the USA. In our opinion, physical examination combined with screening mammography not only can be life-saving for the patient but also may prevent the occurrence of some litigation. On the other hand, sometimes, a skin lesion, sebaceous cyst, wart, hemangioma, or keloid may be projected on mammography as a small mass or causing microcalcification. In the absence of physical examination, the radiologist may request the patient to come back for other useless tests. The radiologist can make the diagnosis of certain affection of breast unknown to a large number of general practitioners, such as chronic infection of seborrhea Montgomery glands, or seborrhea of Montgomery glands, nipple dermatitis, which difficult to differentiate with Paget disease (cancer), nipple bloody discharge during pregnancy, post-pregnancy lactation or breast abscess, breast edema, unilateral or bilateral due to heart failure or vascular obstruction, breast thrombophlebitis, Mondor's disease, breast sclerodermia, coumarin breast skin necrosis, diabetic mastopathy, and pseudo-angiomathous hyperplasia. These are examples that we have noticed in our practice.

It can be argued that if physical examination of the breast is done by the referring health provider, the patient does not need to be examined by the radiologist.

First, I should mention that physical examination of the breast in my experience is excessively difficult. Each patient, at a different age, at a different period of her life has a different shape of the breast at inspection, of different consistency, different firmness at palpation. Cancer manifests clinically each time differently. A breast radiologist has the opportunity to see hundreds of patients and to detect dozens of breast cancer per week by mammography **with different clinical manifestations**. No other health provider has such opportunity to obtain such expertise that the radiologist can get. He or she is in the front line and best suited for physical examination. One of the most important facts is the correlation of physical signs with mammographic findings that are very helpful for diagnosis, which is not in the field of every health provider.

Secondly, many times, several months pass between physical examination by the health provider and the mammography examination. It can happen that clinical sign of breast cancer at that time was very subtle or nonexistent and has developed in the meantime. Common observation is the so-called interval breast cancer; often an aggressive cancer develops clinically and becomes palpable between annual normal physical exam and screening mammography. Mammography may show nothing (20% of palpable cancer cannot be seen on mammography). Thus aggressive cancer can be missed if physical examination is not done. The result of screening mammography can be reported normal.

Thirdly, some physicians are unaware of the weakness of mammography in the detection of all breast cancer and have such a high confidence on mammography that they send their patients for annual screening mammography without performing the physical examination and relying solely on the report of the radiologist. Therefore, physical examination by the radiologist is a necessity. It enhances the efficiency of the radiological profession, and radiologists can be regarded by the public as a real doctor.

Fourthly, now with tremendous advances in technology in medical specialty, a new subspecialty, breast imaging, is born, and the role of breast radiologist in the management of breast cancer becomes prominent and much more responsible. Physical examination of the breast should be an integral part of training in this subspecialty. We definitely need more clinician radiologists—real doctors—than just radiologist breast image interpreters.

MRI OF THE BREAST

One of the most amazing breakthrough in the last century was the discovery of MRI technology (magnetic resonance imaging) and its application in medicine. So far, MRI has saved more lives than any other medical diagnostic imaging. It is unbelievable that by changing electromagnetic polarity of the hydrogen atom of the organ, we can get an image of the entire organ demonstrating the lesion and its function.

How can we detect breast cancer by MRI? By MRI, we can detect not only the anatomy of the cancer but also its dynamic function (speed of the blood exchange). Cancer cells need more blood vessels, forming rapid angiogenesis. Later, it was found that chelated substance with paramagnetic character (gadolinium) enhances the visibility of breast cancer vascularity. Now, it is used currently as a contrast media on MRI examination. We detect the breast cancer on MRI by its hypervascularity (neoangiogenesis).

The patient lies face down on a mobile table. The breasts are placed in holes which contain coils (electronic transmitters and receivers devices). The table is pushed into the tunnel of the large magnet. Pictures are taken from both breasts, then contrast media is rapidly injected followed by injection of saline water. Sixty seconds after the injection of contrast media, again, pictures of the breasts are taken. What we can see in the first series of pictures before the injection of contrast is that cancer image may be seen like a dark black hole, and after injection of contrast media and subtraction of the second MRI series, the black hole turns to a white spot with round or irregular borders representing the anatomy of the lesion. The function and activity of the lesion and exchange of blood in the tumor can be shown by dynamic curve. The more rapid rise and fall, wash-in/wash-out (blood circulation), in the short period of time correlates with the fast-growing lesion, and often cancer biopsy should be performed.

Another variant of MRI is spectrometry by MRI, a technique less used in breast cancer but has higher specificity, because cancer contains high concentration of choline, which can be detected by this technique that can differentiate between benign and malignant lesion.

Breast biopsy by MRI

Breast biopsy under the control of MRI is performed when the lesion is detected only by MRI.

After establishing an IV line, the patient in the same position as above lies face down on a mobile table pushed into the tunnel of the magnet, feet first, then the body and contrast media is injected rapidly followed by saline water, thus the lesion is targeted and the table is pulled out of the magnet, and core needle biopsy can be performed.

MRI is the most effective device to detect small invasive breast cancer. Ideally, it should be used for screening. But because of its high cost, it is not accepted except in limited circumstances. Patients, however, should know about its usefulness, its potential in detection of early breast cancer. At this time, MRI is permitted only on asymptomatic (without complaint) patients who have strong family history of breast carcinoma or are BRC1/BRC2 positive. But we should know that 75% of patients who get breast cancer don't have risk factors or family history. MRI is indicated in the following patients, either with high risk or difficult to detect their breast cancer by mammography:

1. Patients with history of BRC1/BRC2 positive in the family
2. Patients of Ashkenazim ethnicity
3. Patients with strong family cluster of breast cancer in the first/second degree with members of the family having ovarian carcinoma
4. Patients with strong history of fibrocystic breast
5. Patient with strong history of fibrocystic palpable mass in the breast, multiple cyst aspirations, multiple surgeries
6. Patient with dense breasts, numerous surgeries for fibroadenomas, giant fibroadenoma, cystosarcoma phyllodes
7. Patient with implants
8. Follow-up in patients for LCIS, DCIS, and invasive breast cancer
9. Six months after serious trauma of the breast

COMMENTS IN PERFORMING MRI IN BREAST CANCER

1. Because of high sensitivity of MRI, it can detect not only the earliest stage of breast cancer development than any other technique but also any other lesion with more vessels (angiogenesis). Objection is done not only for screening breast cancer because of the high number of false positive, high cost, but also objection is done to MRI when cancer is found in the breast and we want to know if there are additional cancer foci in the breast. In one hundred lesions discovered by MRI, 70% are benign and 30% are malignant. Thus, 70% of the time a biopsy does not reveal cancer. This may cause stress for patients. That is the main argument against MRI. We should ask ourselves: If we

do not do MRI, not causing stress for biopsies, 30% of breast cancer would be missed. But if we do an MRI, we may save thirty lives at the expense of the seventy stressful benign biopsies. Which is better?
2. These objections are not rational. Same objections can be done for physical examinations, for mammography, for ultrasonography. In all these tests between 60% to 80% of biopsies of the lesions detected are of benign nature, then we should not do those tests at all.

Inconvenience of MRI:

1. Rarely allergic reaction to the injection of contrast media gadolinium
2. Claustrophobia in closed MRI
3. Contraindication of injection of contrast media in kidney disease, unique kidney, kidney stones
4. Contraindication of patient wearing or carrying superficial metallic devices
5. High cost

When there is a contraindication of MRI, and there is a necessity to resolve the problem seen only on mammography, patient may have nuclear test for the breast (PET scan).

OUR OBSERVATIONS

It is reported that the size of cancer found by MRI is larger than the size of cancer removed by surgery and in pathology. We should pay attention to the fact that imaging of cancer by MRI represents mostly its vascularity. In laboratory animals, graft of cancer in hamster cheek caused intense hypervascularity, hyperhemia, and hemorrhagic foci around the graft, representing peritumoral angiogenesis; it is the same in the human. In our experience, several cases of breast cancer with intense hypervascularity around or slightly distant from the cancer mass corresponded to the fast-growing and fast-recurring cancer, in particular triple negative or HER2-positive breast cancer. This may not be a good warning sign of the outcome of breast cancer.

In many occasions, we detect DCIS on mammography confirmed by core needle biopsy followed by MRI, which showed more abnormal foci proven by biopsy to be small invasive breast cancer in the same breast or in the opposite side. Even in retrospect, on reviewing mammography, those 6 to 8 mm lesions could not be seen. Mammoprint (genetic test) of some of those cancers showed to be high risk for metastasis. Without MRI these cancers would have been classified as DCIS whereas in reality they should have been classified as invasive breast cancers. This misclassification has a great impact on the epidemiology of national breast cancer registry and on statistical annual incidence of DCIS, thus also making dubious the result of the randomized and nonrandomized trial on DCIS, because these patients did not have an MRI before treatment. Literature shows that when DCIS recurs, in 50% lesions are invasive. We really don't know whether DCIS has turned to invasive breast cancer or invasive breast cancer was present at that time, not detected before treatment, because the patient did not have an MRI. Misclassification has a great impact on the treatment of cancer. DCIS does not need chemotherapy; invasive cancer needs it. Without MRI cancer can be under- or overtreated.

Example of the importance of MRI:

This forty-eight-year-old patient had left outer quadrant DCIS surgically removed with clear margins. Subsequent MRI showed (fig. 8.9) small highly suspicious mass in the inner quadrant of the left breast, not visible on previous mammography. Biopsy showed 6 mm invasive breast cancer. Mammoprint showed high risk for metastasis (giant dwarf cancer). These are examples of harms of not doing MRI: (1) Invasive breast cancer would have been missed. (2) Case would be misclassified as DCIS. (3) Patient would have been undertreated. High risk for metastasis in this young patient requires chemotherapy regardless of the size of cancer.

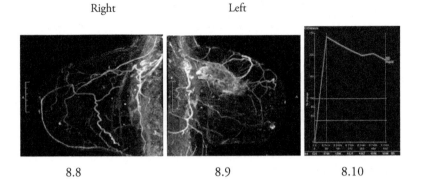

Right   Left

8.8   8.9   8.10

Large white image on the left side is post-surgery for DCIS; small hot spot red color is invasive breast cancer which was not visible on mammography.

Dynamic curve of invasive breast cancer; wash-in/wash-out, typical in cancer

COMPARISON MAMMOGRAPHY AND MRI FOR DETECTION OF BREAST CANCER

MAMMOGRAPHY	MRI
X-ray exposure, carries risk	No x-ray, no risk
Difficulty of cancer detection in dense breast	No difficulty of cancer detection in dense breast
Cannot picture the entire anatomy of the breast	Can picture the entire anatomy of the breast
Often missed tumor less than 5 mm in size	Often detected breast cancer less than 5 mm
Sensitivity of mammography to detect invasive breast cancer in 36%	Sensitivity of MRI is 81% in invasive breast cancer
Detects breast cancer 3 per 1,000 patients	Detects breast cancer 11 per 1,000 patients
More technologist dependency	Less technologist dependency
MAMMOGRAPHY	MRI

Weakness in detection of fast-growing cancer Weakness in detecting invasive breast cancer	Strength in detecting interval and fast-growing and invasive breast cancer
Strengths in DCIS detection	Weakness in DCIS detection
Weakness in detecting recurring breast cancer	Strength in detecting recurrent breast cancer
Interpretation is extremely difficult	Interpretation is much easier
Long learning curve, lifetime experience	Short learning curve
Shows only anatomy of breast cancer	Shows anatomy and physiologic activity of the breast cancer
Cannot show thoracic metastasis	Shows thoracic metastasis
Cannot show lesion in other organs at the same time	Can show lesion in other organs at the same time, e.g., lung, liver
Cheap tool for screening breast cancer	Expensive tool for breast cancer screening
Best trap for lawsuit of missed breast cancer—bad for patients and career devastating for radiologists	Best anti-trap, life-saving for patients and career-saving for radiologist

Despite the weakness of mammography in detecting invasive breast cancer, its strength is shown in detecting DCIS better than any other technique. Overall, mammography can change the modality of the treatment, by comparison of previous mammography. Aggressiveness and progression of the lesion can be assessed, which is often neglected by physicians who are focused only on morphology and pathology (microscopic examination) of breast cancer and not on its dynamics demonstrable by imaging technique. It should be considered as another prognostical predictor, which has never been taken into consideration by treating physicians.

ULTRASONOGRPAHY OF THE BREAST (ECHOGRAPHY)

Ultrasonography consists of scanning the breast with a probe called a transducer which contains a crystal with piezoelectric characteristics which emits mechanical sounds (ultrasound) when an electrical current is applied to it; thus ultrasound waves are directed to the breast through the transducer and, after hitting the interfaces of the breast tissue, bounce back to the transducer. The changes of the waves can be transformed to images and displayed on the screen of a monitor for obtaining pictures. This is the best way to differentiate a cyst containing fluid with solid mass; the solid mass may be benign or malignant, which can be diagnosed by core needle biopsy.

For comparison:

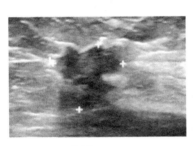

8.11
Irregular dark image on ultrasonography is consistent with malignancy.

8.12
Typical image of benign cyst—oval black image with regular borders, hyperdense (white) posterior border.

INDICATIONS

1. When any patient comes with a palpable mass at any age, first ultrasound should be performed.
2. In any dense breast tissue shown by mammography, ultrasound would help the detection of the nonvisible breast cancer on mammography.
3. Sometimes, cancer is missed on first-time ultrasonography but seen on MRI. In repeated ultrasonography (second

look) focusing on where MRI has shown the lesion more than 60%, the lesion can be found and makes possible core needle biopsy under the control of ultrasonography, which is easier and cheaper than under the control of MRI.

GALACTOGRAPHY (DUCTOGRAPHY): Visualization of milk gland by injection of contrast media

In the young generation of radiologists, two important tests in breast cancer detection are neglected. One is the physical examination, and the other is ductography. They rely mainly on ultrasound and MRI. The importance of physical examination despite all imaging technology was described in the previous chapter. Ductography, when done correctly, is simple, painless, inexpensive, and excessively informative.

INDICATION: Spontaneous, serous, or bloody discharge from one pore of the nipple is suspicious for malignancy. First mammography should be performed. If mammography is negative, then we proceed to galactography instead of ultrasonography or MRI, which are more time-consuming and more expensive. The most common cause of nipple bloody discharge is benign tumor (papilloma) behind the nipple. Sometimes, without ductography some surgeons proceed to useless blind surgery in the hope of finding a papilloma. If no papilloma is found, a breast cancer distant to the nipple may be present but will be missed.

TECHNIQUE: A few millimeters of contrast media (containing iodine) injected via special metallic cannule introduced into the oozing pore and the injection is continued until the patient feels pain, then the injection should be stopped and proceed to do mammography in two directions, which shows opacified duct, either normal (fig. 8.13) or abnormal duct (fig. 8.14). The advantage of ductogram is not only that it determines the exact localization of the lesion, but also sometimes, nipple discharge is caused by the benign fibrocystic condition or a mild chronic inflammation; contrast media by iodine disinfects the duct and stops the nipple discharge.

A forty-six-year-old patient had spontaneous bloody discharge; physical examination, no palpable mass; mammography, dense breast; ultrasonography not conclusive. Only ductography shows numerous lesions proven to be cancer (fig. 8.14).

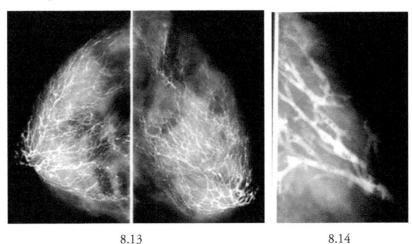

8.13

Normal image of milk ducts by ductography; fine branches of milk ducts in white color

8.14

Ductal cancer, ducts dilated, irregular walls, minute multiple filling defect like small holes (small tumors)

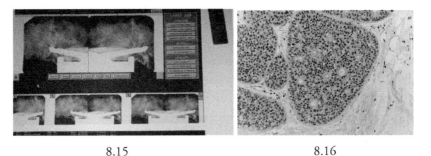

8.15

Stereotactic core needle biopsy after ductography, same patient as in figure 8.14 (technique not published in the literature)

8.16

Specimen removed by core needle biopsy showed cribriform DCIS

RADIONUCLEAR IMAGING IN BREAST CANCER

Images are obtained by a machine similar to the mammographic unit. Pictures are taken after the intravenous injection of radioactive material. Radioactive material accumulates preferentially in the breast cancer tissue, which are then detected by gamma ray detector. There are two different nuclear breast imaging techniques. One is called sestamibi (BSGI scintimammography breast specific gamma imaging; the material injected is radtioisotope technetium 99m). This material injected is uptaken by the mitochondria of cancer cells—source of energy. The other technique is called positron emission mammography (PEM; material injected is radioisotope 18 FDG—fluorodesoxyglucose). Breast cancer is avid for sugar/glucose. Image of cancer can be seen as a bright spot like on mammography. These techniques are not used for screening because of the radioactivity. However, they are used in certain circumstances. For instance, MRI shows multiple lesions in the breast. Multiple core needle biopsies are not practical; therefore, PEM can determine which lesion is more specific to be biopsied. The best way to detect distant metastasis is PET/CT scan combining two techniques together, positron emission tomography (PET) and CT (computed tomography); PET demonstrates hypermetabolic lesion, and CT determines the exact site and location of the distant metastasis.

Conclusion: We describe in detail the failure, weakness, and strength of each modality used for breast cancer detection. If we believe that detection of the small (earlier breast cancer) impacts on survival, then we have to use annual physical examination, annual mammography, and MRI for the general population, which is unaffordable for any nation because of the high cost, unless cost is decreased. Our guideline for breast cancer screening is described in chapter 17.

CHAPTER 9

HOW BREAST CANCER IS DIAGNOSED

BIOPSY OF THE BREAST

Any suspicious abnormality found in the breast either by palpation or by imaging technique should be diagnosed, and it is done only by biopsy.

Diagnosis of breast cancer is done on the specimen of the lesion by the pathologist under microscope. Today diagnosis of invasive breast cancer and its outcome can be determined by genetics study of cancer cells by microarray technique. There are four types of biopsies:

1. FINE NEEDLE ASPIRATION (FNA). This consists of introduction of the fine needle to the lesion and makes vacuum aspiration to obtain cells from the breast. If the lesion is not palpable, aspiration is done under the control of ultrasonography. If fluid is withdrawn and it is clear and the lesion disappears totally after the aspiration, it is consistent with a simple cyst; no further action is needed to be taken. If fluid is bloody or containing pus, it is sent to the pathologist. If the result of pathology is not atypical or the lesion disappears after the aspiration, no further action is taken. If the lesion does not disappear and cytology is equivocal, we should proceed to core needle biopsy. FNA

(fine needle aspiration) is a fast procedure, cheap, with excellent diagnosis for cysts but less accurate and more difficult to diagnose cancer because of a large number of false negative.

2. CORE NEEDLE BIOPSY. The biopsy is done with local anesthetic by special large needle which cuts multiple pieces of the breast tissues. If the lesion is seen only on mammography, the biopsy is done under the control of mammography, called stereotactic core needle biopsy, or if it is seen better on ultrasonography, the biopsy is performed under the control of ultrasonography. If it is shown only by MRI, it is done under the control of MRI. The specimen is therefore sent to the pathologist. The core needle biopsy is a longer procedure, more expensive and more accurate than fine needle aspiration.

3. PUNCH BIOPSY WITH SPECIAL SIMPLE DEVICE. After local anesthesia, by scratching superficially the tissue of the skin by a special device, a specimen can be obtained and sent to the pathologist. This is the simplest way to diagnose between inflammatory breast carcinoma and mastitis (breast infection).

4. OPEN SURGICAL BIOPSY. A big chunk of the lesion is taken by surgery. It is the most accurate for diagnosis. It is the most expensive and done in the operating room with local or general anesthesia. In general by biopsy not only we can make diagnosis of breast cancer, but also before treatment we will have vast information about the outcome of breast cancer, called prognosis.

CHAPTER 10

TRADITIONAL TREATMENT OF BREAST CANCER

In breast cancer, first treat the mind before the body (Charles Gros 1963). A female with a good life, healthy, high-spirited, enthusiastic, courageous, all ends up in a second after learning the result of her cancerous breast biopsy; the whole scenario changes. The healthy patient becomes sick, high spirit wipes out; for hours she goes into a total blackout. She feels highly disappointed, discouraged, overrun by apprehension, anxiety, fear of death, remembering all the sad history about the side effects of chemotherapy—skin and mouth lesions, loss of hair, losing the breast—worrying about the future of her children, and a hundred others. Furthermore, after treatment of breast cancer, chronic anxiety, fear of cancer cells left behind, and breast cancer recurrence continue tormenting the patient's mind on how to cope with all these misfortunes.

All can be remedied to a large degree with compassion; cure mind with heart. Psychological consultation unfortunately is often neglected. If we can provide peace of patient's mind, we have achieved half of the treatment. The patient should know that breast cancer is more innocuous than she thinks; it is very common. Autopsy of females age twenty to fifty who died in car accidents showed 18% had breast cancer (DCIS); patients were completely unaware of their presence. This number would be much higher if autopsies were done in females between sixty to ninety years old. We should convince patients by evidences that all breast cancers are not lethal. A large number of patients die of other causes than breast cancer after a long life.

Patients should know that the variety of local treatment of breast cancer has no impact on survival. Cancer cells may still be present in the body after removal of breast cancer by surgery without any harmful consequences. In the worse scenario with worst prognostic elements, patients have lived more than twenty-five years after surgery of breast cancer without radiation and without chemotherapy. Nobody and no test can tell how long a patient will live after the treatment of breast cancer. Don't rely on statistics and don't rely on prognostic predictors because none of them is valid individually.

TREATMENT OF THE BODY

Today treatment of breast cancer is based on the age, ethnicity, socioeconomic availability of the treatment, psychology of the patient, and histochemistry of the lesion.

On TNM classification, nonresectable cancer undergoes mastectomy; resectable lesion gets conservative treatment. We should always bear in mind to "do no harm." Now we are going to see if we respect our oath with classical treatment of breast cancer.

A. SURGERY: MASTECTOMY

Le Martyre des Croyantes Bib. Nat. Paris

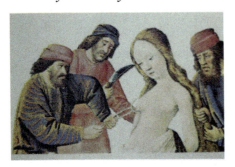

Surgery of the breast has been practiced for thousands of years earlier with primitive tools. Mutilation of the breast was done in barbaric manners. Breast was transfixed with a metal ring then quickly cut away with a sharp knife, then cauterized with fire sticks or with vitriolic acids. It certainly carried high mortality because of uncontrollable bleeding, local infection, and general septicemia. This treatment continued till the eighteenth century with advances in sciences (introduction of general anesthesia in 1868). Microscopic examination of the tissue, discovery of x-ray, and radium transformed the surgical treatment of breast cancer. In 1883 Halsted proceeded to remove the entire breast and all axillary lymph nodes called radical mastectomy. But the cancer continued to come back either to the chest wall or to the thoracic lymph nodes. Surgeons thought the larger surgery would improve the results. Sugarbaker and Urban proceeded to remove the breast by much larger surgery, called extended or super-radical mastectomy, removing the entire breast, both pectoralis muscles, axillary, thoracic, and intramammary lymph nodes, and subclavian lymph nodes. Again, the cancer came back. In Europe, in 1930, Patey with less drastic surgery called modified radical mastectomy reported the same result as radical mastectomy. He proved that with less surgery it is possible to obtain the same result as a large surgery. In 1943, McWhirter from England introduced a new technique, much smaller surgery called partial mastectomy and breast radiation, which reported the same result as radical mastectomy. In

1960, Bacless in France, with high dose of radiation alone, could obtain acceptable results in nonoperable breast cancer leftover of surgeons and demonstrated that mastectomy is not always necessary. Fisher in the USA by randomized trial called B0-4 (1971–1985) and B0-6 (1976–1983) showed the following:

1. Lymph node dissection of the axillae has no impact on survival.
2. Any type of local treatment of breast cancer—radical mastectomy, lumpectomy with radiation, lumpectomy without radiation—had the same survival. As lumpectomy with radiation cuts the local recurrence in half when compared with the lumpectomy without radiation, it becomes the standard of treatment of operable breast cancer. Today, mastectomy consists of the removal of the entire breast, sometimes including a few lymph nodes from the lower part of the axilla, without removing any chest wall muscles unless they are involved with cancer.

CLASSICAL INDICATION OF MASTECOTMY

1. Mastectomy is done for men's breast cancer.
2. In women, mastectomy is done for any invasive breast cancer or DCIS.
3. Mastectomy is done after neoadjuvant chemotherapy in inflammatory breast cancer.
4. Mastectomy is done in multicentric breast cancer.
5. Mastectomy is done for breast necrosis due to the radiation therapy.
6. Mastectomy is done in induced radiation cancer—angiosarcoma.
7. Mastectomy is done in any local recurrence after conservative treatment with radiation.
8. Mastectomy is done in breast tuberculosis or parasitosis.
9. Mastectomy is done in high-risk BRC1/BRC2.
10. Mastectomy is done in Ashkenazim ethnicity with hereditary damaged genes.

11. Mastectomy is done in breast cancer, unilateral or bilateral upon the request of the patient for psychological reasons.

ADVANTAGES OF MASTECTOMY

1. Definitive treatment of DCIS preventing the occurrence of invasive breast cancer.
2. In invasive breast cancer, prevention of outbreak and ulceration to the skin.
3. Prophylactic mastectomy in BRC1/BRC2 which reduces the lifetime risk of cancer from 85% to 5%–10%. A patient with one-sided breast cancer requests bilateral mastectomy for the peace of her mind; this is beneficial. Another case: for a young patient who has to live another thirty to forty years after diagnosis of her breast cancer and who is not willing to undergo such a long time to uncertain tests and follow-ups and thinking and believing that no more cancer will remain in her body and no more cancer can reoccur, bilateral mastectomy is also advantageous.

DISADVANTAGES OF MASTECTOMY

1. Shocking at first to accept such a harsh treatment.
2. Wound infection, cellulitis, or abscess.
3. Seroma and hematoma, which always occur, may delay the healing of the wound.
4. Arm edema, swelling of the arm occurring in 25%, call lymphedema of the arm.
5. Decreased shoulder mobility.
6. Phantom breast syndrome; about 50% of patients after mastectomy complain of pain, itching, nipple sensation, erotic feeling, and premenstrual breast soreness.
7. Disturbance of sexual activity, trouble with clothing, unpleasant body image particularly in young women. Majority of these inconveniences can be dissipated in time or mainly by surgical breast reconstruction.

Two different techniques of mastectomy

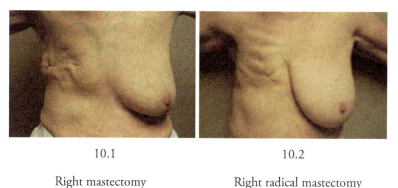

| 10.1 | 10.2 |

Right mastectomy   Right radical mastectomy

B. AXILLARY LYMPH NODE DISSECTION IN CONSERVATIVE TREATMENT OF BREAST CANCER

Axillary lymph node dissection is still an integral part of the surgical treatment of breast cancer when axillary lymph node is involved with metastasis. In olden days, in breast cancer, axillary lymph nodes, palpable or not palpable, were removed as much as possible of the three levels of axillary lymph nodes. It was thought that involved axillary lymph nodes were sources of cancer dissemination and also could have an impact on survival. Test of time has proven otherwise. In a BO-4 randomized clinical trial, 1,559 patients with breast cancer with no clinically palpable axillary lymph node (performed in 1971 to 1985) were divided in three groups. Group 1 had radical mastectomy with lymph node dissection and showed 40% lymph node metastasis in the axilla. Group 2 had total mastectomy without lymph node dissection but had axillary x-ray radiation. Group 3 had total mastectomy but no axillary lymph node dissection and no radiation. That means in this group, 40% of involved lymph nodes was left behind without treatment. The result after eight years, group 1 had 5% lymph node recurrence in the axilla, group 2 had 5% lymph node occurrence, and group 3 had 18% lymph node recurrence. But the most important finding was that **the survival in the three groups were similar** despite the fact that in the third group, about 40% of involved lymph nodes were left behind without treatment but only in 18% did lymph node metastasis recurred, which did not have impact on survival. It should be mentioned that when breast cancer spread metastasis via lymphatic or blood channels, they can involve thoracic, cervical, axillary, intramammary, and abdominal lymphatic nodes. For instance, when the cancer situated in the inner quadrant of the breast with axillary lymph node metastasis in 50%, metastasis are present in intramammary lymph nodes which are not removed. Therefore, by any type of surgery, the knife of the surgeon cannot hunt all involved lymph nodes; lymph node surgery is a ghost-chasing scenario. Therefore, even after lymph node dissection, we should not think that the patient is cleared from lymph node metastasis; 25%–50% of lymph node metastasis that is usually left behind may or may not manifest as recurrence during the lifetime of the patient. All this trial indicates that lymph node dissection in breast cancer is unnecessary (except compressing other structures). Most important, lymph node dissection has no impact on survival.

Breast lymphatic network

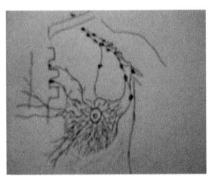

10.3

With such a rich lymphatic network, lymph node dissection with the intention of clearing the patient of lymph node metastasis is more wishful thinking.

SIDE EFFECTS AND COMPLICATIONS OF AXILLARY LYMPH NODE DISSECTION

1. Hematoma, collection of bleeding after surgery in underarm pit

2. Infection
3. Motor nerve damage of the arm
4. Numbness in the axilla and in the upper part of the arm
5. Frozen shoulder, disability of shoulder movement
6. Arm edema, most disturbing side effects

C. SENTINEL LYMPH NODE SAMPLING (BIOPSY)

Because of serious side effect and complication of axillary lymph node dissection and sometimes unnecessary surgery because no lymph node metastasis was found, surgeons resorted to the lesser traumatic and more rational procedure called sentinel lymph node sampling in the axilla (Juliano). This is examined microscopically, instantaneously (frozen section) in the operating room, then if positive, proceeding to axillary lymph node dissection.

Sentinel or sentinel nodes are situated in the lowest part of the axilla, close to the breast tissue. In 90% of the time, sentinel lymph nodes are first involved with metastasis before the other nodes if cancer is in the outer quadrants. Today, sentinel lymph node sampling is practiced in conservative treatment. It is done for prognostic purposes. If it is involved with metastasis microscopically, it leads to axillary lymph node dissection and indication for chemotherapy. Negative sentinel lymph node does not rule out involvement of other lymph nodes. It should be mentioned that sentinel lymph node sampling alone does not totally eliminate complication such as infection or arm lymphedema. There is also 20% of false positive: a few epithelial cells found in the lymph node are due to the biopsy of the breast releasing cancer cells, not real metastasis but may lead to overtreatment, unnecessary axillary lymph node dissection, and chemotherapy. Also, 10% false negative, which means cancer cells bypass sentinel lymph node and involve the upper echelon of lymph nodes. As axillary lymph node dissection has no impact on survival, it has lost its value, and it is considered unnecessary.

D. CONSERVATIVE TREATMENT OF BREAST CANCER: LUMPECTOMY PLUS RADIATION THERAPY

Lumpectomy was an appropriate term in olden days, because all breast cancers at that time were found with lumps. Today, it is a misnomer because a large number of breast cancers is detected before being a palpable lump. Standard of conservative treatment, in invasive breast cancer, is excision of the lesion and sentinel node sampling; if the lymph node is involved with the metastasis, lymph node dissection, then the patient undergoes chemotherapy and breast irradiation. If breast cancer is smaller than 1 cm and no metastasis in the axilla, no chemotherapy but the breast gets irradiation.

In conservative treatment in DCIS, there is no precise guideline. Some surgeons remove the DCIS and perform sentinel lymph node sampling if they find some cells, then lymph node dissection follows. Some patients may be treated as invasive breast cancer.

Some other surgeons remove only the DCIS with or without prior MRI, no lymph node sampling, and the patient may or may not undergo radiation (depending on the size of DCIS).

PROCEDURES USED FOR CONSERVATIVE TREATMENT OF INVASIVE BREAST CANCER

Today, the majority of operable breast cancer are diagnosed by core needle biopsy, and after core needle biopsy, in some institutions, MRI of the breast is performed, then the patient is scheduled for conservative treatment if MRI shows no other suspicious lesion. The day of surgery, thirty minutes before surgery, 0.5 cc of radioactive material (sulfur technetium 99 m) is injected to the skin of the breast, close to the site of the previous core needle biopsy. This is done for targeting the axillary lymph node for biopsy. Also, before surgery, the radiologist, under the control of mammography, introduces a hook wire, a metallic wire, into the breast, directing to the cancerous lesion, called needle localization of the lesion. With this needle, the patient is transported to the operating room. (This needle is to guide the surgeon to remove nonpalpable breast cancer.) Five minutes before surgery, a dye called blue methylene is injected under the skin at the same site of core needle biopsy. This blue dye is transported via lymphatic channels to the axillary and colors sentinel lymph nodes in blue; the surgeon first removes the cancerous lesion in the breast, then with gamma counter finds the lymph node and removes the blue-colored lymph nodes. Once they are removed, they are examined immediately under microscope by the pathologist. If the lymph node is involved with metastasis, the patient undergoes axillary lymph node dissection of level 1 and 2, then followed by chemotherapy and radiation of the breast. As we mentioned before, axillary lymph node dissection has no impact on survival, already abandoned by many surgeons.

E. RADIOTHERAPY OF THE BREAST

When I started medicine in France in 1947, for my training, I was assigned to Curie Institute in Paris. At that time, radiotherapy was the panacea used as penicillin given to all types of ailments. The danger of radiation causing cancer was not well known. We treated diseases such as hemangioma of the skin, birthmarks, eczema, lupus, psoriasis, pruritis, arthritis, degenerative arthritis, arthrosis, back pain, alopecia (tinea capitis), vitiligo, apnea, mastalgia, fibrocystic breast, big thymus in children, goiter, lishmaniosis, leprosis, and chronic wound; in some cases it really worked miraculously well. Later, we learned that x-ray can cause cancer; radiotherapy in noncancerous lesion was interrupted and limited to the treatment of cancerous lesion.

Today, radiotherapy is done in the following cases:

- In conservative treatment, for breast cancer DCIS and stage I and II invasive cancer
- In post-mastectomy for cancer larger than 5 cm
- In post-mastectomy for chest wall metastasis of recurrences
- In post-mastectomy for inflammatory breast cancer
- Radiotherapy for distant metastasis

THE PURPOSE OF BREAST IRRADIATION

Radiation of the breast is performed with x-ray or gamma rays. The purpose of radiation is to kill cancerous cells and prevent the local recurrence. Cancer cells as well as normal cells with fast division like lymph node cells, bone marrow cells, hair follicles, gastrointestinal mucosa, white blood cells are more vulnerable to x-rays than cells with slow division. It took more than half a century to find the optimum x-ray dose to kill preferentially cancerous cells (cancerocidal doses). They tried first with low dose of 300 roentgen, but the cancer came back locally. The dose was then increased to 9,000 roentgen (Curie Institute). Sometimes, the breast was virtually incinerated, necessitating mastectomy. Finally, international dose of 5,500 rad (55GY) was accepted as the optimum dose.

Radiation is given five days a week for five to six weeks.

The benefit of radiation is that it cuts the local breast cancer recurrence in half in conservative treatment when compared with no radiation to the breast. Despite all progress in radiation therapy, side effects and collateral damages and local recurrences cannot be avoided.

COMPLICATIONS AND SIDE EFFECTS OF BREAST IRRADIATION

Why can radiotherapy cause side effects and damage other organs close to the target? It is because X or gamma rays are not like laser beam monochromatic, single wavelength light emitted in direct line hitting only the target. X-rays generated by a source (x-ray tube) are polychromatic; different wavelengths are spread out in all directions and by collision to any atom in the air or to any object nearby generate secondary x-rays. In the radiotherapy of the breast, not only the target (breast) is hit by x-ray and absorbs the highest amount of x-rays, but also adjacent organs such as the heart, the lungs, the liver, and to a lesser extent, the whole body absorb x-rays, which can cause damages. The same mechanism happens in any radiotherapy or by any x-ray machine. See figure 10.4 (a).

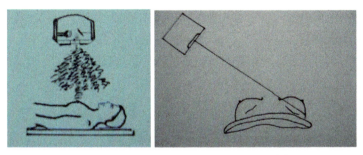

| | Indirect irradiation of the breast |
10.4   10.5

These pictures show that with all artifices, collimation, indirect irradiation of the breast cannot avoid irradiation of other organs (fig. 10.4).

THE SIDE EFFECTS ARE GENERAL, LOCAL, REGIONAL, AND DISTANT, REPORTED IN THE LITERATURE IN THE WHOLE BREAST IRRADIATION.

General is the fatigue during the treatment.

Local complications and side effects in the breast itself:

1. Acute effect during the radiation therapy consists of inflammation of the skin, redness, and erythema with wet desquamation.
2. Long-term protracted redness, peau d'orange, breast edema.
3. Irradiation-induced highly lethal breast cancer angiosarcoma, 1 out of 470 cancers, ten to fifteen years after the treatment.
4. Mastectomy because of extensive radiation necrosis and infection.
5. Because of intense changes of breast structure, fibrosis and scar, recurrence in at least 30% of breast cancer cannot be detected by mammography and detected by large mass on palpation.

Regional side effects and complications of breast cancer with whole breast irradiation:

1. Radiation pneumonitis six to eighteen months after radiotherapy, cough, shortness of breath, fever.
2. Fibrosis, scar of a portion of the lung, chronic dry cough, shortness of breath.
3. Pleural effusion, cough, shortness of breath, back and chest pain, fever.
4. Increased cardiac death five to ten years after treatment.
5. Increased lung cancer, latency about ten years, incidence of 9 per 10,000.
6. Irradiation increases the risk of congestive heart failure after chemotherapy.
7. Arm lymphedema 7% to 30% of the patients.

Distant side effects and complications of breast cancer by irradiation:

1. Acute nonlymphocytic leukemia four to seven years after the treatment.
2. Cognitive problem similar to chemobrain. It can last for years after breast cancer treatment with radiation.

In the last decade, because of the serious side effects of the whole breast irradiation and unavoidable loco regional tissue damages inducing also other types of cancer, we have resorted to lesser amount of irradiation to the breast by a technique called brachytherapy, which irradiates only parts of the breast at the site of the cancerous lesion. In brachytherapy, several techniques have been used. One is called mammosite, which consists of inserting a bag containing small radioisotope particles emitting gamma rays into the cavity created after the removal of cancerous tissue. The bag containing iridium 192 is replenished twice a day for five days, delivering 3,400 cGY. Another technique is <u>intraoperative x-ray therapy;</u> while the patient is in the operating room, after removal of the breast cancer, still under general anesthesia, a special cylindrical-shaped x-ray tube is put in contact with the tissue at the site of the removed cancer, and irradiates to 2,000 cGY one time. This technique seems to be very attractive because of no general side effect; however, there are inconveniences that have not been emphasized.

1. No information of the margin if residual cancer left behind, intraoperative frozen section for margin assessment has no role in the pathology for diagnosis of DCIS (Lagios).
2. Longer procedure in the operating room.
3. General anesthesia.
4. Leaving local fibrosis, scar, fat necrosis, impeding the detection of local recurrences.
5. Local side effect, chest wall bone necrosis.
6. Much costlier than simple excision and no radiation.

PERSONAL OBSERVATION OF PATIENTS FOLLOWED DURING AND UP TO TWENTY-FIVE YEARS AFTER CONSERVATIVE TREATMENT, LUMPECTOMY, AND RADIATION THERAPY OF THE WHOLE BREAST

1. Skin changes, erythema, redness, thickening, orange peel (peau d'orange), edema, discoloration, telangiectasia, shrinkage, fibrosis, keloid may persist twenty-five years after treatment.
2. Pain and tenderness persist in some patients for twenty-five years.
3. Thrombosis of subclavian artery occurred ten years after radiotherapy of the right breast cancer. First case not reported in the literature.
4. In some patients, damage to the breast tissue continue over twenty-five years, progressive fibrosis, fat necrosis, new appearance of microcalcifications, new appearance of masses leading to numerous core needle biopsy with no cancer.
5. In several cases because of breast tissue fibrosis, recurrent cancer could not be detected by mammography until it becomes palpable. We observe in many cases, the original cancer was 1.5 cm, nonpalpable; recurrent cancer was diagnosed when it was 3.5 cm and palpable.
6. Cosmetically, shrinkage of the breast started soon six to nine months after completion of radiation. Patients surviving twenty-five years without exception had moderate to excessive shrinkage.
7. In several cases, noticeable progressive shrinkage of the breast was thought to be of radiation fibrosis, but mastectomy revealed diffuse recurrent breast carcinoma, not diagnosed before the surgery (first case reported in the previous author's book published in 1996).
8. Arm lymphedema after sentinel lymph node sampling and breast irradiation.

Side effects of radiation in the treatment of breast cancer in different patients and different ages, twenty-five years after irradiation

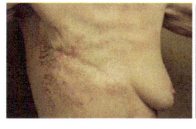

10.6

Post-mastectomy radiation, telangiectasia, abnormal vascular formation

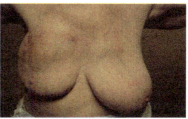

10.7

Right post-lumpectomy radiation shrinkage, discoloration, telangiectasia of both breasts due to scattered radiation

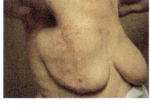

10.8

Right post-lumpectomy radiation, telangiectasia

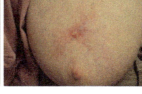

10.9

Left post-lumpectomy radiation, keloid formation at the incision of the breast

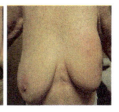

10.10

Left post-lumpectomy radiation shrinkage, breast discoloration

The following cases, post-lumpectomy, radiation, photo of some patients with their respective comparative mammography with the opposite side shows unsatisfactory deformity, retraction, fibrosis, and hyperdensity, which impede early detection of breast cancer recurrence.

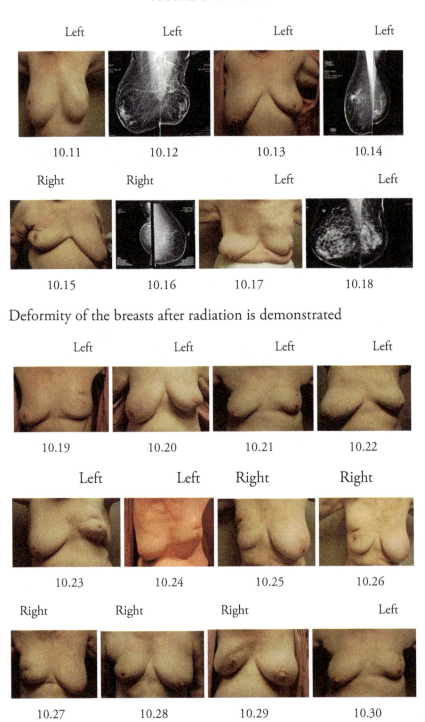

Deformity of the breasts after radiation is demonstrated

FIGHT NEW WAYS BREAST CANCER

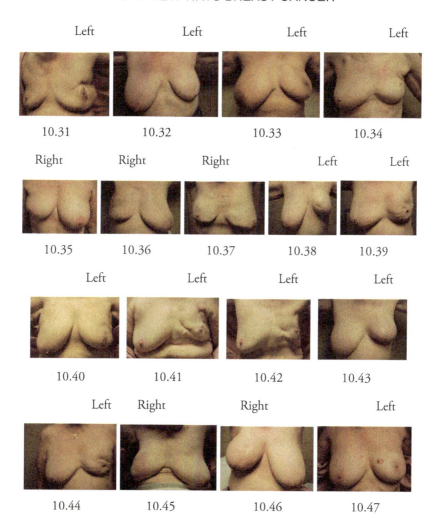

Right	Right Left
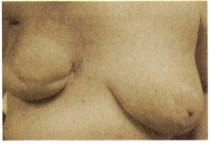	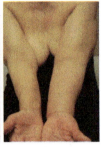
10.48	10.49
Right breast reconstruction after conservative treatment radiation therapy, recurrence mastectomy	Left arm edema 2 years after axillary sentinel lymph node sampling and breast irradiation

THE RESULT OF INVASIVE BREAST CANCER IRRADIATION VERSUS NO IRRADIATION

Four international randomized trials, comparisons of survival of patient who had irradiation of the breast versus no irradiation were done on over four thousand patients by the American, Swedish, Canadian, and Italians. None of them showed significant survival benefits in patients who had irradiation therapy of the breast versus no radiation.

In 2000 (Lancet), the early cancer trialist collaborative group published meta-analysis of ten and twenty years of result from 440 patients of randomized trials of radiotherapy for early breast cancer, showing reduction of 2% to 4% mortality in twenty years in favor of radiation. But if we take into account cardiovascular mortality in that group, we find the absolute gain of radiation was only 1.2%, statistically insignificant.

In 2007, in *The New England Journal of Medicine*, Dr. Hughs reported, in 621 women aged seventy, node-negative with breast cancer of 2 cm, no benefit of breast irradiation over Tamoxifen alone on survival. A Canadian study published in the same issue including younger women age fifty and older found irradiation of the breast had no impact either on distant metastasis or on survival. In Orebro's (Uppsala) trial, women aged over fifty-five, cancer size less than 2 cm, who had surgery alone (lumpectomy) had 11% recurrence in ten years with surgery and radiation 6.1%. The authors concluded that radiation is unnecessary, as twenty women should be irradiated in order to prevent one case of breast cancer recurrence, which has no impact on survival.

REPORTED RESULTS OF IRRADIATION IN THE TREATMENT OF DCIS VERSUS NO IRRADIATION

Because DCIS has been epitomized noninvasive cancer, lesser research and lesser randomized trial have been done than for invasive breast cancer.

In 1993 NASBP (National Surgical Adjuvant Breast Project) published the result of prospective randomized trial between two groups of patients with DCIS (describe previously); in one group, excision of DCIS then post-surgical radiation, the other group excision alone without radiation. In the group without radiation the local recurrence was twice than the group with the radiation, but survival statistically was not different. Despite that, disregarding the side effect of radiation therapy, lumpectomy and radiation therapy were advocated as the treatment of choice of DCIS. Subsequently, two other international randomized trials, one by EORTC (European Organization for Research and Treatment of Cancer) and the other by UK/NZ and one nonrandomized trial (Silverstein), showed no survival difference between the two groups.

Strongest clinical and pathological predictors in DCIS was published by our group called Van Nuys prognostic index (VNPI) in 1996 (Dr. Silverstein).

Pathological Criteria: Size of the DCIS score (1 to 3), nuclear grade (1 to 3), clear margins (1 to 3), presence or absence of intraluminal necrosis.

If DCIS had a total score of 3, the lesion was considered as a low risk for recurrence; therefore, excision alone without radiation was appropriate.

Total score of 5 to 7 was considered high risk for local recurrence; excision plus radiation more suitable.

Total score of 8 to 9 was considered higher risk for local recurrence; mastectomy was the treatment of choice.

The latest report by Dr. Silverstein et al. based on 1,000 patients with DCIS, 644 treated with excision alone and no radiation and 356 treated with excision and radiation, showed 30% recurrence of DCIS without radiation and 17% with radiation. Invasive recurrence without radiation was 37% and with radiation was 57%, statistically significant, but the reason is unexplained.

Survival at ten years in nonirradiated breast was 99.7%, better than irradiated breast, 98.3%.

Two important findings in this report were the following:

1. Time of recurrence in DCIS nonirradiated breast was two years after the diagnosis; in irradiated breast it was four years.
Invasive breast cancer recurred four and a half years after treatment of DCIS in nonirradiated breast and on irradiated breast seven years later. Radiation neither cures nor prevents breast cancer but postpones its recurrences.
2. In nonirradiated DCIS invasive breast cancer occurred in 9% in other quadrants versus 26% on irradiated breast—statistically significant but the reason is not explained. It might be due to the fact that more harmful and more extensive DCIS underwent irradiation where some more foci of DCIS or invasive breast cancer were present and undetected.
Or induced x-ray breast cancer cannot be ruled out.

If the outcome of DCIS is measured by its recurrence, irradiation of the breast is twice more effective than excision alone without irradiation, but if the outcome is measured by survival, irradiation of the breast has no impact on survival, even slightly better without irradiation.

Conclusion: In olden days we thought that radiation of the breast could cure breast cancer. That is why we see in old textbook that irradiation of the breast was divided in two parts—curative radiation and palliative radiation of the breast cancer. Curative radiation connoted for a small breast cancer thought curable, and palliative for advanced ulcerated nonoperable and incurable breast cancer was done to heal its ulcerations. Time proved that breast irradiation is neither curative nor preventive. The only apparent benefit is the reduction in half of breast cancer recurrence, which has no impact on survival. All these facts should be presented to the patient before instituting breast irradiation. Here we reported cosmetic side effects and damages caused by irradiation of the breast despite all sophisticated procedures used in the USA, such as simulator machine, computer dosimetry, supervoltage, linear accelerator, and electron boost. Damages are much higher in a large part of the world where they do not have those sophistications. Nonetheless, patients are treated with irradiation for breast cancer; thus, no radiation is better than radiation.

CHAPTER 11

SYSTEMIC TREATMENT OF BREAST CANCER

Systemic treatment of breast cancer consists of chemotherapy and anti-hormone therapy. Breast cancer can be totally eradicated from the breast; it does not need systemic treatment. Chemotherapy is done only for cancer cell metastasis in the blood, in the lymph nodes, or grafted into the other organs. Chemotherapy uses toxic chemical substances, called cytotoxic, that by toxicity kill normal and cancerous cells with fast division. Cytotoxic drugs prove curative in some cancers such as chorioepithelioma of the uterus, germ cell cancer, acute lymphoma, leukemia, sometimes of non-Hodgkin's lymphoma, and testis cancer.

Chemotherapy is efficient in fluid type of cancer cells such as cancer cell in the blood in the bone marrow. It is much less efficient in solid type of cancer such as in breast cancer. Chemotherapy has been based on findings, on randomized trials (NSABP) and Italian, which showed at ten years in treated groups, 51% of patients were alive, and in nontreated, 45%. The difference was only 6%.

In 2005 (Lancet), early breast cancer trialist collaborative group, Oxford analysis was published with chemotherapy in patients less than fifty years old; at fifteen years, mortality was 32.4%, with and without chemotherapy 42.4%. The difference was only 10% reported benefit. Chemotherapy in patients more than fifty years old, at ten years, mortality was 47.4%, with and without chemotherapy, 50.4%. The difference was that 3% reported as benefit of chemotherapy.

Most chemotherapy used today is AC = doxorubicin 60 mg/m^2 + cyclophosphamide 600 mg/m^2 every three weeks for four cycles. TC = taxane 175 mg/m^2 + cyclophosphamide three weeks for four cycles.

A. INDICATION OF SYSTEMIC TREATMENT OF BREAST CANCER (CHEMOTHERAPY)

Classic systemic treatment of breast cancer is based on clinical predictors, size of tumor larger than 1 cm and positive axillary lymph node, age of patient, and comorbidities (other disease).

If chemotherapy is done after removal of the breast cancer either in conservative treatment or after mastectomy, it is called adjuvant chemotherapy. If it is done before surgery, it is called neoadjuvant chemotherapy. It is done mainly in inflammatory breast carcinoma or large palpable breast cancer. The purpose and the hope of this procedure is to debulk cancerous lesion, and the patient may be switched from mastectomy to conservative treatment, also a test of efficiency of the medication and a justification for continuation of the same medication. In any large non-inflammatory breast cancer, genetic test of the cancerous lesion should be performed in order to determine which cancer is more sensitive to chemotherapy and which cancer is more sensitive to anti-hormone therapy.

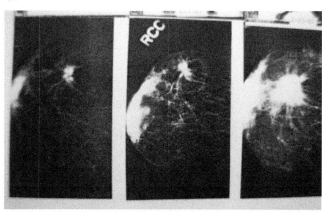

11.1	11.2	11.3
6 months after chemo	3 months after chemo	start of chemotherapy

This 53-year-old patient had chemotherapy for palpable large cancer (fig. 11.3). Chemotherapy debulked cancerous lesion (white crab-shaped image) to a small nodule (fig. 11.1), and the patient switched from mastectomy to conservative treatment, preserving her breast.

SIDE EFFECTS OF CHEMOTHERAPY

Cytotoxic substances not only kill cancerous cells but also any fast-dividing cells in the body such as hair follicles, causing hair loss; bone marrow cells, causing myelodepression and anemia; and gastrointestinal cells, causing abdominal pain, loss of appetite, nausea, vomiting, diarrhea, mouth sores, and mucositis.

Cardiovascular toxicities, acute cardiac toxicity, pericarditis, fever and chest pain, congestive heart failure, chronic cardiopathy, pain, swelling and redness in hands and feet (hand and foot syndrome), hemolytic anemia, infection, neurotoxicity, neuropathy, peripheral edema, fluid accumulation, transitory infertility (young patient), or permanently in perimenopausal status, chemobrain syndrome, osteoporosis, bone fracture—chemotherapy has created a new branch of medicine which takes care in treating its secondary side effects. In fact, by the classical chemotherapy we intoxicate one hundred patients in order to obtain at best 10% to 20% survival benefits, no benefit for 80% of patients. If we base our chemotherapy on genetic tests, we will get better results (chapter 15).

PUBLISHED COMMENTS ABOUT EFFICACY OF CLASSIC CHEMOTHERAPY OF BREAST CANCER:

Craig Henderson, oncologist, in a textbook (*Breast Diseases*) said: There is as yet no empirical evidence for clinical study that any group of patient is cured with adjuvant chemotherapy who would not have been cured with local treatment alone and this applies as much to node negative patient as to node positive patient.

Skipper et al.: If chemotherapy incapable of curing overt metastases might well be capable of curing microscopic metastasis.

Rojagapal et al.: Surveyed 307 American and European oncologists. They were asked to state the benefit of chemotherapy, which was published by EBCTCG analysis found that oncologists overestimate the remission by chemotherapy **by twice** the actual percentage and improvement of survival **by three times** the reported value. Oncologists are overly optimistic about the benefits of chemotherapy. This misconception is commonly presented to patients, which may influence them to undergo chemotherapy that in their cases cytotoxicity with all side effects is not needed.

MODERN SYSTEMIC BREAST CANCER THERAPY BASED ON GENETICS OF CANCER

These consist of immunotherapy, monoclonal antibody therapy, target therapy, ongoing nanothechnology, and nanoparticles therapy.

Immunotherapy: In our body white blood cells, mononuclear, polynuclear, and B and T cells are responsible to defend us against bacteria, virus, and cancer. Mononuclear and polynuclear recognize bacteria as foreign bodies, attack them, and destroy them. White T cells, natural killers, do not recognize cancer cells because they are from themselves. Cancer cells, however, produce protein (antigen); we can use it against them. T cells of patients are embedded with their cancer cells in the laboratory; thus protein called antibody is formed in the T cells, which make the T cells capable of recognizing cancer cells, attacking and destroying them. Specific antibody proteins can be used against breast cancer, called monoclonal antibody therapy, such as Herceptin used in breast cancer, which contains abnormal amount of protein called HER2. Recently researchers have found another reason why T cells can't attack cancerous cells. That is because of a brake, the presence of a protein called PD1 in T cells. Now by inhibiting the activity of PD1 (check point inhibitor) by specific medication, a monoclonal antibody (Yervoy) blocking that brake, T cells attack and destroy cancer cells. It is used in triple-negative (estrogen, progesterone, HER2) breast cancer, with most effective result.

Ongoing new systemic chemotherapy in cancer, called nanooncology, was reported in CANCER; in this technique, the nanoparticle (one billionth meter), organic material such as liposome (fat) or inorganic material such as metals, gold, iron coated with chemotoxin, antibodies or silencing DNA substance, is injected to the bloodstream. This material, nanoparticles, after getting out of the vessels, penetrate easily into cancerous cells. There, toxic or killing substances are unloaded and causing the death of cancer cells, or nanoparticles inside the cells can be irradiated by low energy, near infrared light or laser beam. By hitting metal, light energy converts to heat up to 45 centigrade, creating a real furnace inside the cells and incinerating cancerous cells. The result of such a therapy is waiting.

According to the genetic discovery of breast cancer, the mission of metastatogenicity is established in the molecular stage. However, we do not know exactly when the spread of metastatic cells start. We don't know either of the sequence of the spread of metastasis; is it constant or intermittent? But we know that as cancer grows, the number of metastasis increases as well. Therefore, it is important to detect breast cancer as small as possible if it is in high risk for metastasis, we assume that lesser number of metastasis is spread, therefore more vulnerable to chemotherapy than when large number of metastasis is grafted in the body. It is important to know which cancer is in high risk for metastasis before discovering the metastasis. Today, it becomes possible by genetic test mammaprint in invasive breast cancer.

Four types of breast cancer are designated by genetic test, which lead to target therapy:

1. Cancer called luminal A, characterized by estrogen receptor and progesterone positive and HER2 negative. Proven to be low risk for metastasis less than 10%, comprising 40% to 60% of invasive breast cancer. Treatment: surgical excision, no need for lymph node status, no need for chemotherapy, eventually Tamoxifen in premenopausal and Arimedex in post-menopausal if tolerated by the patient.

2. Cancer called luminal B, characterized by estrogen receptor positive, progesterone receptor low or negative, HER2 negative, comprising 30% of breast cancer. If genetic test shows low risk for metastasis, treatment is similar to luminal A; if high risk, patients are treated with anti-hormone and chemotherapy. Recently, new medicine (ibrance) has been reported to be efficient in post-menopausal patients with distant metastasis .

3. Cancer called basal, characterized by estrogen and progesterone receptor, and HER2 negative (triple negative), comprising 15% of breast cancer, high risk for metastasis, treated with chemotherapy, and recently monoclone antibody (Yervoy) in metastatic triple negative has provided good survival benefits. This cancer is very sensitive to chemotherapy, sometimes long remissions after three initial violent upheaval years after the diagnosis have been observed.

4. Cancer called HER2 positive, high risk metastasis, chemotherapy and antibody (Herceptin) are indicated, comprising 15% of breast cancer. It should be noted that genetic test for low risk or high risk is based on study of seventy genes of cancerous cells whereas determination of subtype of breast cancer is based on eighty genes. Some nasty subtype such as triple negative or HER2 positive are in low risk. Theoretically they don't need chemotherapy, but at this time no oncologist accepts that risk without randomized trials.

In conclusion, the result of classical chemotherapy in breast cancer is modest; at best, favorable response is only in 25% of patients. We do not have any better means to treat or prolong life eventually to cure the patients. Right now, chemotherapy is going to be based on genetics signature of molecular subtype. It has already changed the practice, result yet unknown. We hope we will get better results than classical chemotherapy.

B. HORMONE THERAPY AND ANTI-HORMONE THERAPY IN BREAST CANCER

<u>Hormone therapy:</u> As strange as it can be, hormones such as estrogen, progesterone, testosterone have been used against breast cancer over half a century, still prescribed in very advanced breast cancer, sometimes with good and long remission as was said before.

The paradox is that, in one hand, hormones, particularly estrogen, are reputed to cause breast cancer; on the other hand, they are used against breast cancer for its treatment.

<u>Anti-hormone therapy:</u> Chemical substances such as Tamoxifen, a carcinogenic substance (causing cancer of the uterus), is used against breast cancer. Tamoxifen acts only on certain breast cancers, in those cancers that their cells contain hormone receptors in their surfaces. It is postulated that Tamoxifen, by blocking hormone receptors, stops the cancer cells from capturing hormones from the blood for its metabolism, therefore can cause their death.

Tamoxifen 20 mg a day is used mainly in premenopausal females. Another chemical substance called Arimedex is used 1 mg/day in post-menopausal women. In post-menopausal women, there is no production of estrogen from the ovaries, but the adrenal glands secrete testosterone. An enzyme called aromatase exists in the breast tissue but mainly in the fatty tissue of the body, which can transform testosterone to estrogen. Arimedex has the capability to inhibit the function of aromatase; thus cancer cells are deprived of estrogen. Tamoxifen, Arimedex, Aromasin, and Femara are from the same family, called selective estrogen receptor modulators (SERMS).

CLINICAL TRIALS FOR ADJUVANT TAMOXIFEN THERAPY

To date more than forty randomized trials have been performed in order to access the effectiveness of adjuvant Tamoxifen in breast cancer—20 mg per day for five years. The result reported as follows:

1. Tamoxifen prevents the recurrence of breast cancer in 50% and prolongs survival in 7% in patients whose breast cancer has estrogen receptor positive and lymph node involvement (stage II).
2. Tamoxifen used in breast cancer with receptor positive or negative with negative axillary lymph nodes, shows no benefits.
3. About 60% of breast cancer in post-menopausal women are estrogen receptor positive and 40% in premenopausal patients.
4. 60% of breast cancer with estrogen positive are responsive to Tamoxifen.
5. The more cancer cells contain estrogen receptor positive, the more responsive to Tamoxifen.
6. Tamoxifen does not impact on survival of patient with DCIS.

THE CLINICAL TRIALS IN ANTI-HORMONE THERAPY AS PREVENTIVE MEDICATION

Four randomized trials for accessing the effectiveness of Tamoxifen in high risk-patients for breast cancer were done, one in the USA and three in Europe. Randomized trials (NASPB) in healthy patients with high-risk factors for breast cancer, age more than sixty, Gail test more than 1.7, strong family history of breast cancer, show the following:

1. A group of patients who took Tamoxifen for five years developed 2.2% cancer . The group that did not take Tamoxifen for five years developed 4.3% cancer . Relative risk reduction was 49%, but in reality absolute risk reduction was 2.1%.
2. It was shown that Tamoxifen was efficient in preventing invasive breast cancer in patients with LCIS and in ductal hyperplasia.
3. Tamoxifen was not efficient in preventing breast cancer in healthy women carrying BRC1 and BRC2 positive.

4. Authors of the trial recommended Tamoxifen in preventing breast cancer with high-risk factor of the general population. Tamoxifen as preventive drug was tried in England and in Italy in high-risk patients and did not find the same result and the same benefit, but they found all the same toxic side effects of Tamoxifen that was found in the American trial.

SIDE EFFECTS OF TAMOXIFEN FOUND IN RANDOMIZED TRIALS

Despite the fact that NASPB excluded women with cardiovascular risk and no exclusion was done in placebo group, they noticed the following side effects:

1. Risk for pulmonary embolism was three times higher in the group with Tamoxifen.
2. Risk for thrombosis was three times higher with Tamoxifen.
3. Risk for stroke was two times higher with Tamoxifen.
4. Hot flashes were two times higher with Tamoxifen.
5. Vaginal symptoms, discharge, dryness, and itching were much more with Tamoxifen.
6. Ocular toxicity, intraretinal crystals, and cataract were more with Tamoxifen.
7. The most serious side effect was the carcigenicity of Tamoxifen, increased risk of endometrial cancer (uterus). With Tamoxifen it was 5% whereas in placebo it was 2.3%. Relative increased risk of the cancer of the uterus is 260%.

Patients on Tamoxifen should have continuous, regular gynecological examination and uterine ultrasonography. Any progressive thickening of the uterine walls requires biopsy so as not to miss uterine cancer.

In NASPB, the danger of endometrium cancer was minimized, but Holland suggested that unlike NASPB, mortality is greater than average. That means that provoked uterine cancer by Tamoxifen is more aggressive and more lethal than uterine cancer of ordinary female population.

Authors of the trials in Italy and England did not recommend Tamoxifen as preventive medicine in healthy women.

Gail and others emphasized that despite major reduction risk of 50% in all subgroups in breast cancer trials and accepting the results as "truth," use of Tamoxifen in selective healthy women at increased risk is usually a close call, that the benefit and the risk is marginally different.

Side effect of Arimedex: Suppression of aromatase increases the risk of osteoporosis, thromboemboli, cardiovascular disease, urogenital atrophia, vaginal bleeding, and other types of toxicity of Tamoxifen as well.

C. NEOADJUVANT ANTI-HORMONE THERAPY

Recently anti-hormone therapy has been tried before surgery in large breast cancer. After core needle biopsy and confirmation of breast cancer and the presence of estrogen receptor positive by genetic test, using anti-hormone may cause shrinkage of the tumor of the breast, and then patients may get conservative treatment instead of mastectomy.

In conclusion, anti-hormone therapy as adjuvant medication has modest benefits. The patient may take it despite its serious side effects. In healthy women, as preventive medication, it is very questionable. Therefore, before prescribing anti-hormone therapy, the benefits and side effects of the drug should be explained in detail to the patient. The patient will make conscious decisions. Example, Rush Port reported the result of an interesting research from Memorial Sloane Kettering Cancer Center in New York, interviewing forty-three high-risk patients aged less and more than fifty years with a Gail 1.7% history of LCIS. Once they explained the benefits and the risk of side effects of Tamoxifen, only 2% accepted to undergo treatment with Tamoxifen as a preventive medication. It should be known that prolonging the duration of remission by drug is not without toxicity and has only a minimal effect at best on overall survival.

CHAPTER 12

BREAST CANCER RECURRENCE

Breast cancer can reoccur locally in the breast, regionally in lymph node of the chest wall, and distantly in other organs after any type of treatment of breast cancer.

1. Local recurrence: Breast cancer can recur after mastectomy with or without previous chest wall irradiation. These recurrences are metastatic cancer stage IV, most likely hematogenic, harbinger or concomitant to a general systemic metastasis, and may start by small subcutaneous nodule appearing often on a scar line of previous mastectomy. If these nodules are not treated, more nodules appear and gradually break out, ulcerating to the skin, bleeding, getting infected with bacteria or fungus, and finally putrefaction, septicemia, fever, and death. There is another type of chest wall cancer recurrence seen after mastectomy with irradiation—gradual redness, extensive thickening, hardening of the skin like an armor plate, called breast cancer en cuirasse, appearing on the entire hemithorax with ominous outcome. Treatment consists of extensive surgery of the chest wall. Prognostic often unfavorable.
2. Breast cancer recurrence after conservative treatment, so-called lumpectomy, with breast irradiation: 80% of breast cancer recurs at the site of previous resected cancer if primary breast cancer was detect by microcalcifications

on mammography. When it recurs, it manifests again by the same type of microcalcifications. If the primary cancer was detected by mass on mammography, it recurs often and appears as a mass on mammography. If the primary cancer was negative on mammography and cancer was detected by palpation, often it recurs the same way. Classic treatment is mastectomy. Prognostic often favorable.
3. Regional breast cancer recurrence: Breast cancer can recur after any type of treatment, enlarging lymph nodes in the axillae, lateral to the sternum (intramammary lymph nodes), in the neck, compressing adjacent tissues. Treatment is with surgery and radiation therapy and chemotherapy. Unfavorable.
4. Distant metastasis in organs such as lung, liver, bones, and visceral. Treatment is with surgery and radiation and chemotherapy. Unfavorable.

Here, we emphasize more on the recurrence of breast cancer after conservative treatment of breast cancer with radiation.

Causes of local breast cancer recurrence:

1. Cancer is removed without clear margin (majority of recurrences), cancer cells left behind.
2. Cancer is removed surgically with clear margins, marginal cells left behind if examined under microscope, morphologically are normal but they may be mutated genetically and later develop to cancer cells, and cancer recurs (mutation of the genes cannot be seen by microscope).
3. Cancer was originally multifocal or multicentric, not detected before surgery as reported before. Today, we know, with MRI, a large number of multifocality and multicentricity or bilaterality can be detected before surgery. In the past, in randomized trials, MRI did not exist. Therefore, we do not know exactly how many of the

recurrences were due to preexistent multifocality or multicentricity of breast cancer.
4. Radiation despite the maximum dose fails to destroy all breast cancer cells, or cancer cells probably originated from stem cell, which is resistant to irradiation, or maximum dose was not enough to destroy this residual marginal cancer.
5. We know that x-ray by itself is a high risk to induce breast cancer as well, example given in the previous chapter. Maybe some recurrences are due to x-ray-induced breast cancer.

In conclusion, in the absence of MRI before surgery, we cannot know if the development of the recurrence is due to a new breast cancer or preexistent, undetected breast cancer.

Can we prevent breast cancer recurrence?

According to the literature in conservative treatment, about 50% of surgeries for breast cancer are repeated because at first attempt clear margins could not be obtained, some residual left behind. The surgeon re-intervenes a second and third time in order to get cancer tissue out with clear margins. It should be said that before the first surgical attempt, by needle localization, it is possible to target the lesion, or the marker deployed by core needle biopsy of the lesion, the surgeon is guided to remove the cancerous lesion. But in the second or third time the lesion cannot be localized because there is no marker; it is removed by previous surgery. The surgeon intervenes blindly in scar tissue, removes a large amount of the breast, which has two inconveniences. First, at each attempt, removing more breast tissue causes more scar tissue and more breast deformity. Second, even when the tissue is removed with clear margins, there is no guarantee that no cancerous tissue is still left behind. The main reason of the failure to obtain clear margins at first-attempt surgery is in nonpalpable breast cancer, the radiologist localized the lesion only by single hook wire; with one wire, the lesion cannot be removed totally. In

1982, when we started hook wire localization biopsy in our comprehensive breast center, we had the same problem. Then the author initiated to introduce two to four hook wires around the lesion in order to bracket the entire lesion, since that time exceptionally second and third interventions were necessary. Good surgery depends on the exact localization and removal of the entire cancerous lesion at first surgical attempt after doing MRI. The entire resection of the lesion with clear margins and excellent cosmetic results depends on the experience of the radiologist and expertise of the surgeon on oncoplasty surgery of the breast.

As was said in conservative treatment of breast cancer, the majority of recurrence is due to residual cancerous tissue left behind. Numerous publications have shown that larger breast surgery such as quadrantectomy caused lesser recurrence, but the larger surgery provoked more breast deformity; therefore, we should try with focal surgery to get enough clear margin and preserve the breast with good aesthetic aspect. Good surgery of the breast with clear margins is not always easy. Breasts are of different size, different shape (small, medium, large, gigantic), and pendulant with different consistencies (fatty, soft, dense, hard, rock hard). In fact, the breast is a bag containing mobile, soft, malleable tissue. Excision of cancer is not like scooping out a well-rounded ball from inside of a watermelon. Sometimes, the breast tissue is so hard that it cannot be cut off by a scalpel; other times, there are more problems with pendulant, rolling breasts. On the other hand, cancer to be excised is localized by radiologist only with one needle. That is why the whole cancer cannot be excised. Radiologists and surgeons should have spatial imagination for needle localization and removal of breast cancer. Bracketing technique that we initiated since 1982 can alleviate many of the above problems.

OUR TECHNIQUE

We have been using needles with hook wires. The breast is immobilized and compressed on mammography table by a plastic plate that has an open graduated window (fig. 12.3) through which needles can be inserted from the skin, closest to the lesion, twelve o'clock lesion from the top; for the underneath lesion from six o'clock, in order to bracket the entire lesion, two to four needles or more are inserted 1 cm away from the border of the lesion seen on mammography. Most of the time, still clear margins cannot be obtained because needles inserted during the compression of the breast move backward when the breast is decompressed, and breast tissue stretches out, the entire cancer lesion cannot be removed. In order to prevent that, the needles should be inserted at least 2 cm behind the posterior border of the lesion. By bracketing technique, it is possible to reduce the recurrence from 14% to 2% when combined with post-biopsy MRI (Greg Senofski).

The norm, 1 hook wire   Our technique, bracketing technique more than 2 wires

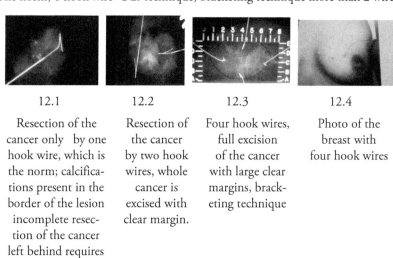

12.1	12.2	12.3	12.4
Resection of the cancer only by one hook wire, which is the norm; calcifications present in the border of the lesion incomplete resection of the cancer left behind requires reintervention.	Resection of the cancer by two hook wires, whole cancer is excised with clear margin.	Four hook wires, full excision of the cancer with large clear margins, bracketing technique	Photo of the breast with four hook wires

Technique for ductectomy not reported in the literature: Ductal lesion is found by ductography—immediately after ductography, irregular duct spotted and numerous hook wires introduced all along the sick duct. The surgeon, with a longitudinal incision, removes the entire abnormal duct.

Craniocaudal projection   Lateral view, needles inserted 1 cm behind the sick duct

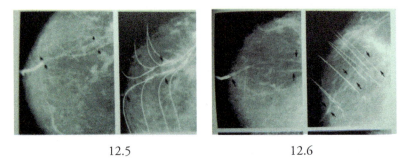

12.5   12.6

Patient had right bloody discharge. Mammography and ultrasonography were inconclusive. Ductography showed proximal obstruction of the duct (arrows), distal irregular duct faintly opacified with contrast media (arrows, fig. 12.5). Hook wires were inserted in each side of the sick duct, and the entire duct was removed surgically, proved to be micropapillary ductal carcinoma. Two extremities of the duct were free of malignant cells.

THE MEANING OF LOCAL BREAST CANCER RECURRENCE OF THE CONSERVATIVE TREATMENT

In the last century, breast cancer was diagnosed too late, often ulcerated with more than 70% lymph node metastasis. Not long after mastectomy, metastasic nodule appeared in the subcutaneous chest wall, getting infected and, as we mentioned before, finally leading to septicemia and death. This is the memory that physicians had from the notion of local breast cancer recurrence. But today local breast recurrence of early breast cancer after conservative treatment has a different meaning. Still, some physicians think that the recurrence in conservative treatment of breast cancer can be an instigator of a new source of metastasis; that is why they precipitously proceed to mastectomy. Despite the fact that in 1999 (Lancet journal), Fisher, et al., following patients of BO-6, published: "Significance of Ipsilateral Recurrence of Breast Cancer Treated Conservatively." Their conclusion was that when breast cancer recurs, risk of distant metastasis is three to four times greater. This is a powerful independent predictor of distant metastasis while mastectomy and breast radiation prevent expression of this marker. **They don't lower the risk of distant metastasis. These treatments might be considered inappropriate.** Breast cancer recurrence is not an instigator of new sources of metastasis, but it is an indicator of worse outcome, therefore no impact on survival. It should be mentioned that randomized trial BO-6 was done on palpable breast cancer up to 4 cm in size, including a large number of advanced cancer in today's standard, most likely with many microscopic distant metastasis. This is why it was found that the risk of distant metastasis is three to four times higher with breast cancer recurrence. Standard treatment of breast cancer recurrence after conservative treatment is still mastectomy.

Today is different with new concept of breast cancer which is based on its genetic signature; the meaning of breast cancer recurrence and its treatment has been totally changed. Local recurrence of breast cancer usually originates from residual cancer cells, genetically similar to the original breast cancer. The risk of distant metastasis and the outcome are not determined by the local breast cancer recurrence. It is defined by its genetic signature before recurrence. However, in any local breast cancer recurrence, genetic test should be performed. If original cancer was in high risk for distant metastasis, local recurrence has no impact on survival, but if original cancer was in the low risk and local recurrence is in high risk for distant metastasis, then it can impact survival. The patient needs systemic chemotherapy. By new ways of breast cancer treatment, if the recurrence is resectable, still the breast can be preserved and not always mastectomy.

CHAPTER 13

MALE BREAST CANCER

Breast cancer in males is rare and represent less than 1%; in women, 99%. The cause of breast cancer like in women is unknown. A man with a female close relative with breast cancer is at high risk; the risk is higher than in general population. Risk factors in men are testicular abnormalities, infertility, breast trauma, persistent gynecomastia, and genetic hereditary disease such as Klinfelter. Approximately, 20% of men with breast cancer carry a genetic mutation of BRC2. A man with genetic mutation can pass it to his offspring; therefore, a man with breast cancer should have a genetic test or genetic counseling. Because of lack of awareness of breast cancer in men, diagnosis is made late, often large tumor with axillary lymph node metastasis. Men who notice a lump or nipple bloody discharge should have a mammography. The majority of breast cancer in men are found behind the nipple; in women, more at the periphery of the breast. In men, often the cancer developing behind the nipple is mistaken for gynecomastia, which is a benign lesion. This is breast tissue behind the nipple which can be stimulated by drugs, blood pressure medication, hormones released by the pituitary gland, or testicular tumor, forming a mass behind the nipple. Treatment of the gynecomastia is to find out its cause. Treatment of breast cancer in men is modified radical mastectomy with lymph node dissection. Some centers advised chemoradiation for large tumors. In men, 90% of breast cancer is estrogen receptor positive; therefore, Tamoxifen for five years is prescribed.

Difference of breast cancer in men and women:

1. Cause of breast cancer is unknown in both sexes.
2. Age: The average age of diagnosis of breast cancer in men is over sixty years old, older than in females.
3. In men, early breast cancer is hardly detected, and when detected, it is by the patient himself. In women, most early breast cancer is detected by mammography or other imaging technique.
4. In men, there is no annual screening mammography; in women, annual breast checkup, mammography after forty.
5. Cancer in men in 20% is BRC1/BRC2 positive; in women, 5% to 10%. Women with BRC1/BRC2 positive have 80% risk of getting breast cancer; in men, 7%.
6. Breast cancer in men in 90% is estrogen receptor positive; in women, 40% to 60%.
7. Treatment of breast cancer in men is always mastectomy; in women, conservative treatment is possible, lumpectomy with or without radiation.
8. Follow-up: In men, there is no special follow-up after treatment of breast cancer; in women, every six months for five years with intense checkup, physical examination, mammography, and other tests.
9. The most important, survival from breast cancer in men is equal to women's survival.
10. Breast cancer treated in men for one hundred years has not been changed (mastectomy); in women, enormous changes have occurred—conservative treatment, oncoplasty surgery.
11. Breast cancer in women has created numerous gigantic industries for society; breast cancer in men, nothing.
12. Publishing industry: Every day, there is something new, in books, magazines, and newspapers about breast cancer. If a thousand-page book about breast cancer is published, 999

pages are dedicated to female breast cancer and only one page to men.
13. Imaging industries: Breast cancer in women created billion-dollar industries for cancer detection, started with film mammography, xeromammography, digital mammography, tomosynthesis, special x-ray machines, breast MRI, high-tech ultrasonography, elastography, nuclear medicine, radioisotope, and breast PET scan; in men, nothing.
14. Radiation industry: High kilovoltage machinery, brachytherapy, mammosite radioisotope, intraoperative one time x-ray radiation, all for women; for men, nothing.
15. Surgical industry: Lumpectomy, sentinel node sampling, reconstruction of the breast, microsurgery, tummy tuck, artificial implant silicone/saline, oncoplasty, all for women; none for men.
16. The latest and newest-born industry is genetics, which will be seen in chapter 15.

Finally, when you consider that survival of breast cancer in men and in women is the same with all this medical backup and gadgets, gain and yield in reality are more for industries than for women.

CHAPTER 14

IS DECLINE OF BREAST CANCER MORTALITY DUE TO OUR TREATMENT?

If we look carefully to the chart of cancer mortality published each year by the American Cancer Society, we realize that the rise and fall of cancer incidence mortality don't always have a plausible explanation like many other diseases in medicine. In the past, there have been back-and-forth epidemic breakouts such as plaque, cholera, syphilis, typhus, EBOLA, which after killing thousands of people go to hiding and remaining endemic. We cannot say why breast cancer in certain individuals in some ethnic minority or in black female is more aggressive and deadlier and why mortality of breast cancer is fluctuating in time.

According to the published data by the American Cancer Society in the matter of cancer:

1. Mortality of uterine cancer declined regularly from 1930 despite no change of its number of incidence, they may explain by using Pap smear of the cervix of the uterus. But this test was universally used since 1954.
2. Mortality of stomach cancer rose from 1930 to 1936 and suddenly declined from 1936 despite no change on annual incidence. This may argue that it was due to the treatment of helicobacter pylori, but that test was applied since 2000.

3. Mortality of colon cancer rose from 1930 to 1945, decline from 1948 up to now. It may argue that's because of colonoscopy and removal of polyp. But this procedure started in 1970.
4. Mortality of lung cancer rose regularly from 1930 to 1968 and suddenly exponentially rose in 2000 then started to decline—no explanation for that. The decline may be argued for the effect of the bans of cigarettes smoking, but it cannot explain sudden exponential rise of mortality in 2000.
5. Prostate cancer, gradual rise of mortality from 1930 to 1948, plateaued from 1948 to 1992, sudden rise from 1994 to 1996, then sharp decline from 1996 with no explanation, PSA was created in 1970.
6. Breast cancer mortality rose regularly from 1930 to 1999 (no explanation) but declined since 1990 despite the fact that annual incidence rose since 1975 and stabilized in 2003. Modest decline of 1.7% annually of mortality of breast cancer is believed to be due to the use of mammography, chemotherapy, and no use of HRT (post-menopausal hormone treatment). In the author's opinion, this decline most likely is due to several factors.

First: Unknown fluctuating factors, rise and fall in cancer mortality in general.

Second: Chemotherapy provided noticeably clinical cure.

Third: DCIS before 1980 counted for 10% to 15%, and in 2010, 30% of all breast cancer of women per year.

Mammographic detection and treatment of DCIS since 1980 most likely largely prevented the occurrence of lethal invasive breast cancer.

Fourth: The importance of mammographic factor; it is reported that in 1970 only 25% of breast cancers were stage I, and in 1980 because of mammography, it reached to 60%.

Mortality of breast cancer before 1980 counted 80 in 100,000, and in 2010, 65 in 100,000 women per year.

All indicate that detection of early breast cancer (DCIS) and smaller invasive breast cancer by mammography had impact on reduction of mortality. However, we cannot rule out lead time bias in the decline of mortality; if after a decade mortality rises, then lead time had a role.

LEAD TIME BIAS

It is believed in the medical community and in the public that detection of small cancer carry longer survival than a large breast cancer. In reality, the survival depends of the aggressiveness of cancer and not on the size. For example, two breast cancer patients with the same aggressiveness, one 10 mm and the other 50 mm, are diagnosed at the same time; the one with 50 mm dies in two years and the patient with 10 mm dies in ten years. Apparently, the small cancer lived eight years longer than the larger cancer, but in reality eight years earlier this large cancer was 10 mm. This eight years is the lead time that the patient has lived before that we don't take into account. In fact, both of them lived ten years.

STAGING OF BREAST CANCER

The purpose of staging of breast cancer is to determine the prognosis and administer appropriate and specific treatment.

For a century, we have been concentrating on knowing the biology of breast cancer by staging, its size, its histochemistry, and genetic signature, which are one side of the story. The other side of the story is human biology, action and reaction against a foreign invader, which are precisely unknown, why a breast cancer with similar biologic characteristics cohabits peacefully with the patient for more than twenty-five years and another one causes the demise of the patient in a few months.

Staging of breast cancer has been developed empirically by surgeons upon their clinical findings. Currently, staging is an international classification based on clinical and pathological findings called prognosticators: size of tumor (T), status of lymph node (N), and presence or absence of distant metastasis (M). TNM classification have been evolved since 1954, initiated by Denoix, a French surgeon. In 2010, complete classification was published by AJCC (American Joint Committee on Cancer), which consists **of fifty divisions and subdivisions** combining different sizes of cancers, different clinical modalities, and different numbers of axillary lymph node involvement with metastasis; presence or absence of distant metastasis makes this classification extremely complex and not applicable. Here, we mention the very simplified version of staging reported in the literature.

Stage 0, intraductal carcinoma in situ (DCIS), survival 98% at ten years.

Stage I, tumor size is less than 2 cm (T1), no lymph node involvement (N0), no metastasis (M0); survival is 80% at ten years.

Stage II, tumor size is between 2 cm and 5 cm (T2), or lymph node involvement (N1), no metastasis (M0); survival is 50% at ten years.

Stage III, tumor larger than 5 cm (T3), or axillary and intramammary lymph node metastasis (N2), no distant metastasis (M0); survival 28% at ten years.

Stage IV, tumor at any size, any lymph node involvement but with distant metastasis (M1); 20% survival at ten years.

Fifty divisions or subdivisions of stages (AJCC) would have been very useful if we had different types of treatments for different stages, but today we can resume our treatments in two acts. (1) Breast cancer is resectable; the patient gets conservative treatment. If not resectable, gets mastectomy. (2) Either one axillary lymph node with metastasis or twenty, we have one type of treatment, which is chemotherapy. The most important issue for us is to know who should get chemotherapy and who should not. This is not provided by TNM classification. Fortunately, recent discovery in genetics of cancer provides us the clue. If we want to compare the genetic test with TNM classification, it should be said that TNM is a classification built in a retrospective manner. We have to remove cancer to determine the size, to do axillary lymph node sampling for status of axillary lymph node; if metastatic, to perform a complete lymph node dissection of the axilla in order to define the number of lymph node involvement and then determine the predictors of prognosis. Genetic test is a prospective predictor regardless of the size of cancer, axillary lymph node status, just on examining genetically the specimen of the core needle biopsy; it can determine who is in the low risk for metastasis and does not need chemotherapy, who is in high risk for metastasis and needs chemotherapy. In addition, only genetic test can determine which protein of cancer is the driver of breast cancer proliferation and treat it with specific medication. None of them is possible with TNM predictors.

PROGNOSTIC OF BREAST CANCER UPON ITS CLINICAL AND HISTOCHEMISTRY

FAVORABLE PROGNOSIS	RELATIVE UNFAVORABLE PROGNOSIS
Age more than 50	Age less than 50
Postmenopausal	Premenopausal
No family history of breast cancer	Family history of breast cancer
No genetic hereditary for breast cancer	Genetic hereditary for breast cancer
No inflammation of the breast	Inflammatory breast cancer
No axillary lymph node positive	Axillary lymph node positive
Cancer DCIS	Invasive cancer
Invasive cancer less than 1 cm	Invasive cancer more than 1 cm
No skin changes	Skin changes, edema, ulceration
Grade I	Grade III
Monocentric	Multicentric

Slow-growing cancer on mammography	Fast-growing cancer on mammography
Punctate microcalcifications	Crushed-stone type of microcalcifications
MRI low dynamic activity	MRI high dynamic activity
Proliferative index KI67 less than 10%	Proliferative index KI67 higher than 10%
Hormone receptor positive	Hormone receptor negative
HER2 negative	HER2 positive

PROGNOSTIC OF BREAST CANCER UPON ITS GENETIC FINDINGS

FAVORABLE PROGNOSIS	RELATIVE UNFAVORABLE PROGNOSIS
Oncotype diagnosis < 10 R Score	Oncotype diagnosis > 40 R Score
Mammoprint low risk for metastasis	Mammoprint high risk for metastasis
Subtype Luminal A	Subtype basal and triple negative
Subtype HER 2 negative	Subtype HER 2 positive

Today, by putting together clinical findings, histochemistry, and genetic test of cancer, not only can we predict more precisely the prognosis and the outcome of cancer, but we can also determine the most appropriate treatment.

CHAPTER 15

GENETIC TESTS IN BREAST CANCER (DECODING BREAST CANCER)

Breast cancer is caused by genetic mutation of breast cells. This mutation of cells may transfer to offspring by parents, causing cancer called hereditary breast cancer; damaged amplified genes are called BRC1/BRC2 positive and exist in all cells in the body. If mutation of breast cells happens during the lifetime after conception causing cancer, it is called sporadic breast cancer. Abnormal genes exist only in the cancerous lesion, not in the cells of the whole body. Currently, three types of genetic test are available.

1. Diagnosis of hereditary breast cancer can be made by genetic test of mouth saliva by swab cotton.
2. Now two genetic tests are performed routinely on cancerous tissue.

These three genetic tests are of paramount importance. They tell us how to prevent or how to reduce the risk of breast cancer and how to treat it. Two genetic tests used routinely in breast cancer tumor are oncotype Dx and mammaprint.

1. Genetic test studying twenty-one genes of cancerous lesions called oncotype DX can determine the risk of local recurrence, and what is more important, it can determine the risk of transformation of DCIS to invasive breast cancer. It is scored 0 to 100; RS (recurrent score) 0 to 39 is

low risk for local recurrence, 39 to 55 is intermediate risk for recurrence, and more than 55 is a high risk for recurrence. RS over 55 translates to 15% to 20% risk for invasive transformation. Low and intermediate risk benefit of conservative treatment, high risk in certain circumstances benefit of mastectomy. In 2012, a group of oncologists (Ben, Solin group) reported in ASCO the results of genetic test (oncotype DX) in DCIS. They found that genetic test was an independent predictor for local recurrence superseding all other clinical and pathological prognosticator. By using this data, now we are able to treat DCIS more appropriately than before.

Example:

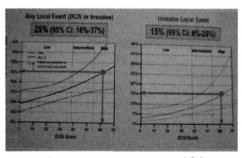

15.1   15.2

In this diagram, the horizontal line represents the number of scores of recurrence, and the vertical line corresponds to the percentage of risk of recurrence. In this patient with DCIS, her recurrent score was 60. It predicted that the risk of recurrence both DCIS and invasive cancer was 25% (fig. 15.1), and the risk of recurrence of invasive breast cancer was 15% (fig. 15.2). Therefore, oncologic workout (MRI of the breast and the body) should be done; if breast cancer is monofocal and resectable and no genetic aberration, patient can have conservative treatment.

Genetic test studying seventy genes for invasive breast cancer, called mammaprint. In 2002 a group of Danish researchers (J. Vande Vijuer et al.) published their work "Gene Expression Signature as a Predictor of Recurrence in Invasive Breast Cancer" in the *New England Journal of Medicine*. Using microarray analysis of seventy genes, prognosis profile on 295 consecutive patients with primary breast cancer, the findings were amazing, and the authors concluded: "Ability of breast cancer to metastasize to distant site is an early and inherent genetic property. This finding argues against the widely accepted idea that metastatic potential is acquired during multiple steps of tumorogenesis, thus an early onset of metastatic capacity theoretically **limits the benefit of early detection and treatment.**"

By this genetic test about 40%–50% of breast cancer is of low risk for distant metastasis with only 10% risk of recurrence in ten coming years, and 40%–60% of breast cancer are of high risk with 29% risk of distant metastasis in ten coming years. These findings are highly important; 40% to 50% of low-risk breast cancer does not need chemotherapy. This test prevents over- and undertreatment of breast cancer which is highly beneficial for patients and financially for the society.

Numerous subsequent publications using seventy genes in breast cancer confirm the original findings of the Danish researchers. Today mammaprint with seventy genes is done to determine the amount of the risk of distant metastasis. When eighty genes are examined, they determine the subtype of breast cancer—luminal A, B, basal, triple negative, HER2 positive. For each type of cancer there are different approaches and different treatments.

15.3	15.4
Classical diagnosis of breast cancer is made on microscopic examination of the tumor.	Modern diagnosis of invasive breast cancer is done by genetics of the tumor cells.

Astonishing facts are that genetic findings today confirm the wisdom of some clinicians of last century. Gershan-Cohen (1950) postulated that the metastatic property and destructive nature of breast cancer are predetermined and inexorable; our interventions do not change the natural history of breast cancer. Mustagalio (1972) from Finland and Fisher (1977) from the USA expressed their views that breast cancer is a systemic disease from the onset. Later in 1999 Kragano et al. showed metastatic cancerous cells in the blood circulation of 95% of early stage of breast cancer, Stage I and II. Sprat, Platkin (1997) from the USA believed that metastasis is spread before we detect breast cancer. Extraordinary findings of the Danish authors unfortunately were not scrutinized by the medical community in more than a decade of their genetic discoveries; their values are not yet recognized, and it is not accepted and applied universally by physicians, except by a few avant-garde oncologists, despite the fact that the test has been cleared by FDA. However, no work has been done to contradict the value of these genetic findings or degrade their importance. In summary, the impacts of genetic discovery in invasive breast cancer are the following:

1. Natural history of breast cancer is led by genetic changes. Different types of mutation in cancer cells cause different behavior. Recent research on prostatic cancer despite low concordance

between genetics of the cell and its microscopic morphology has shown similar mechanism. Prostatic cancer is either low or high Gleason from the onset. Low grade does not upgrade to high grade. If this finding is confirmed universally, it is a noticeable advance in medical oncology. This would prevent multiple biopsies of low Gleason for fear of transformation to high grade.

2. In breast cancer, genetic test can determine either invasive cancer is in low risk or high risk for metastasis. This is a real breakthrough in breast oncology. Breast cancer with low risk for metastasis does not need chemotherapy; high risk, subject to chemotherapy.

3. Thus, genetic test can surrogate lymph node sampling and lymph node dissection because if tests show high risk, chemotherapy is indicated; it is most effective than surgery and radiation therapy. Not only axillary lymph node metastasis but all involved thoracic lymph nodes will be melted away. Even if there remains some residual of metastasis in the lymph nodes, this has no impact on survival. Patient dies of distant metastasis, not by lymph node metastasis. Genetic tests are independent predictors of the outcome of breast cancer, which are far superior than our classical predictors (TNM).

Efficacy of chemotherapy on lymph node metastasis

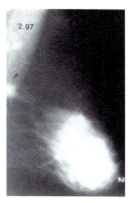
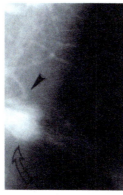
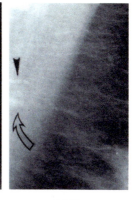

15.5	15.6	15.7
Large breast cancer with axillary lymph node metastasis (arrows)	Magnification of the axillary lymph node metastasis (same patient)	6 months after chemotherapy, surgery of lymph node showed residual fibrosis of lymph node

4. By studying eighty genes of breast cancer, subtype of breast cancer can be determined; for each type, specific medication or target therapy can be used.
5. Genetic studies reveal to us today why in randomized trial of screening mammography in the group of over fifty years there was 25% survival benefits when compared with the group without screening mammography, not only because in screening mammography group smaller-size cancer was found but also because with mammography more cancer was detected, and among them more lowrisk breast cancer for metastasis were present that contributed to the longer survival.
6. <u>How genetic findings can change our practice in management of breast cancer.</u>

Genetic findings in breast cancer show that the outcome of breast cancer is predetermined, in molecular phase before we detect breast cancer; thus, it defies the notion of our early breast cancer concept and utility of screening mammography because sooner or later detection of breast cancer does not alter its ultimate natural history. However, there is a caveat; when we detect small breast cancer less than 1 cm, in 40%–50% this is in high risk for metastasis. If it already had spread metastasis, still they might be in occult stage, which most likely is more vulnerable to chemotherapy than overt metastasis of larger cancer. That is why screening mammography is still strongly advised, particularly for detection of DCIS.

If DCIS is not treated, 30%–40% are potentially invasive breast cancer with 50% mortality. For detection of DCIS, we do not need to use highly sophisticated devices, unaffordable for 9 out of 10 world nation. Simply using the cheapest device, film mammography, which can detect DCIS (microcalcifications), progenitor of invasive breast cancer, by eradication of DCIS, we can eliminate the risk of occurrence of invasive breast cancer. Film mammography is affordable for most poor world nations and is a better device than any others used for DCIS detection. **In the context of genetic concept**, annual physical examination and simple mammography suffice for breast cancer screening. However, as yet, genetic concept is not known and not accepted by a large number of physicians and, by and large, the public, who firmly believe that our early detection of invasive breast cancer makes huge impact on survival. In reality, for detection of small size of invasive breast cancer in general public after the age of forty, we should use breast cancer screening, annual physical examination, digital three-dimensional tomosynthesis, contrasted bilateral MRI, high-tech ultrasonography, and nuclear breast imaging at least for thirty years. This is the price that the patient and society should pay for detection of small breast cancer, unaffordable for any nation. Finally, <u>it is not certain that survival would be better</u> than in genetic screening policy described above. However, as long as the genetic concept is not universally accepted, we have to continue at least screening breast cancer by a compromised policy (chapter 17).

7. Superiority of genetic test over classical prognostical predictors, in invasive breast cancer.

    A. There are 20% to 30% of discrepancy between classical histochemistry of breast cancer and genetic predictors. For instance, in classical histocytology of breast cancer, Grade I is assumed to be very favorable breast cancer. Genetic test shows 20% of Grade I are high risk for metastasis; 20% of patients may get undertreatment. The same is seen in Grade III, assumed aggressive and unfavorable breast cancer by histology, whereas genetically it is demonstrated that 20% of Grade III are low risk. Therefore, this 20% may get useless, harsh treatment of chemotherapy. Same discrepancy is found for HER2 and hormone receptors. Therefore, genetic test is more reliable than classical histochemistry of breast cancer.

B. Genetic test studying seventy genes in Danish research found that spreading metastasis is either lymphogenic or hematogenic—two distinct entities, two different prognoses. In the last century we thought that general spread of metastasis was only via the lymphatic system and the first relay was the axillary lymph nodes, then distant organs. Genetic test shows that the lymphatic nodes may be involved without distant metastasis or vice versa. Distant metastasis is hematogenic origin may be spread through the blood vessels without lymph node involvement. This concept is very important for the treatment.

Example, what to do with a 2 cm breast cancer and two axillary sentinel lymph node involvement with metastasis? Some surgeons go for radical mastectomy plus chemotherapy. A large number of surgeons go for lumpectomy, axillary lymph node dissection, radiation of the breast, and four cycles of chemotherapy. Only very few oncologists obtaining the genetic test of the tumor if it shows low risk go for simple lumpectomy without axillary lymph node dissection, no radiation, no chemotherapy. We cannot imagine the magnitude of psychological, emotional, and economical difference in such cases.

8. Who needs oncological workup during treatment of breast cancer based on genetic tests?

Before genetic findings, we did not have guidelines, how and who should be followed oncologically during or after local breast cancer treatment. Some physicians request indiscriminately whole body CT, PET/CT scan, and nuclear medicine for any type of invasive breast cancer.

Today, genetic test done on core biopsy guides us that only high-risk breast cancer for metastasis need oncologic follow-up, not for all invasive breast cancer, which makes a great impact on nationwide economy.

9. GENETIC IMPACT ON THE NOTION OF EARLY BREAST CANCER

WHAT IS EARLY BREAST CANCER? IS SMALL BREAST CANCER EARLY? EARLY OR EARLIER DETECTION?

The most important factor in breast cancer is to find out its prognosis. Prognosis determines the type of treatment and the outcome of the patient. Prognosis of breast cancer at this time is based on its size; it is believed that small breast cancer is early and is of good prognosis, and as it grows it becomes nastier and nastier. Therefore, cancer size less than 2 cm without axillary lymph node metastasis is called early breast cancer stage I, and sometimes stage II as well. However, there are arguments that small cancer is not synonymous to "early"; 25% of patients with so-called early breast cancer, less than 2 cm (stage I), die in five years despite surgery, radiation, and intense chemotherapy, and 10% of patients with 5 cm of breast cancer live for twenty-five years without radiation and chemotherapy. In fact, 25% of stage I are already stage IV, unknown by notion of early breast cancer. It is not unusual to find a very small size of breast cancer not palpable, not visible on mammography or on MRI but found only on mastectomy done because of palpable axillary lymph node metastasis or elsewhere. Therefore, the outcome of cancer cannot be determined by its size; that is the first argument that small breast cancer is not early biologically. **But it is earlier when comparing the size of 1 cm to 2 cm.** Therefore, we should use earlier breast cancer detection, not early breast cancer detection.

Breast cancer develops in different manners with different aggressiveness.

Two cancers born at the same time, one originates focally from a few milk ducts, the other originates segmentally from a thousand milk ducts, both with the same progression. At the same time, one is detected small, 1 cm (because originally focal), and the other at 5 cm. The smaller cancer is still called early breast cancer despite the same biology and chronology.

Two cancers originated focally at different times. One takes three years to reach 1 cm and the other born later but in a few months reaches 5 cm. The latter is younger, but still the 1 cm is called early breast cancer. The biology of breast cancer cannot be determined by its size; this is the second argument.

Genetically, early breast cancer is when carcinogenic mutation takes place in the cell in molecular stage that we cannot detect cancer at that time, but we can detect genetic mutations long after, when we diagnose cancer in tumoral stage. Only at this time we can determine the prognosis and the outcome of cancer. In DCIS, oncotype Dx determines the risk of occurrence of invasive breast cancer, and in invasive breast cancer mammaprint test defines the risk of occurrence of distant metastasis. Therefore, genetic test determines the prognosis and the outcome of the patient, not the size of cancer. Today, notion of early breast cancer based on its size belongs to the past.

If the physician wants to know about the prognosis of a patient's breast cancer, instead of looking at the pathology report for the size of the breast cancer, the physician should look at the report of genetic test of breast cancer.

In previous chapters, we used in numerous occasions the term "early breast cancer" for small size of cancer despite the fact that small breast cancer represents neither its chronical age nor biological outcome. Nevertheless, we use that term because 60% of small breast cancer is of good prognosis; detection of small breast cancer and expressing it as early, psychologically, is very rewarding to the patient, thinking her cancer has been caught on time.

CONCLUSION: The outcome of breast cancer depends on its genetic signature, not on its size. When we discover a 5 mm cancer without axillary lymph node metastasis, we are very happy believing that the cancer has been caught on time with good outcome, whereas when we discover a cancer of 50 mm with axillary lymph node metastasis, we are very unhappy, cancer caught late with dire outcome. In both instances we are mistaken. The outcome may be reversed; the 5 mm cancer can be fatal in three years, and the 50 mm alive another twenty-five years.

Finally, a small cancer does not mean it is early biologically. Early breast cancer detection should be replaced by earlier (size wise) breast cancer detection.

CHAPTER 16

ALTERNATIVE TREATMENT OF BREAST CANCER VERSUS STANDARDS

Primum non nocere (First do no harm).

"New opinions are always suspect and usually opposed merely because they are not already common knowledge" (John Locke).

First, briefly we mention standard treatment of DCIS and invasive breast cancer based on TNM. Then we discuss and compare with alternative treatment of breast cancer based on genetic findings.

STANDARD TREATMENT OF DCIS

Indication of mastectomy:

"Mastectomy can be performed in any type of DCIS." But empirically we learn that mastectomy is not necessary in all cases of DCIS. The most accurate criteria for mastectomy were presented by our group Van Nuys prognostic index (Dr. Silverstein) but are not practiced universally. Actually, mastectomy in DCIS is performed arbitrarily upon personal opinion of treating physicians. We most likely will get better results if we combine Van Nuys prognostic index with genetic information of the patient and her cancer, which provides more precise indication of mastectomy in DCIS. It leads us to the following:

Alternative surgical treatment of DCIS

We should be reminded that contrary to invasive breast cancer in which a variety of local treatments of the breast has no impact on survival, local treatment of DCIS might have a great impact on survival. Total eradication of DCIS may prevent the occurrence of lethal invasive breast cancer or DCIS with mission of metastasis.

In DCIS, the choice of modality of the treatment depends on the assessment of the risk of occurrence of invasive breast cancer.

1. Patients with genetic test BRC1/BRC2 positive
2. Patients with Ashkenazi ethnicity with genetic aberration of BRC1
3. Patients exposed in young age to high dose of radiation, either accidental (nuclear disaster) or for treatment of thoracic lymphoma

In the above cases the risk of occurrence of invasive cancer is very high; therefore, the most appropriate and rational treatment, the best choice, is bilateral mastectomy with possibility of breast reconstruction.

Patients with genetic aberration should have bilateral prophylactic mastectomy and bilateral oophorectomy as well. The reason is that 70% of ovarian cancer is detected in late stage III or IV. This large surgery reduces the risk of invasive cancer in both areas.

Unilateral mastectomy is the best choice for DCIS in patients with strong family history, clustered invasive breast, and ovarian cancer and recurrent score more than 60 oncotype Dx or score 7–9 Van Nuys prognostic index (Silverstein), or extensive DCIS, DCIS in the entire breast, killer DCIS.

Standard Conservative Treatment of DCIS

"It consists of removal of DCIS axillary lymph node biopsy, radiation of the breast."

Again, conservative treatment of DCIS is practiced arbitrarily; some surgeons insist on removal of DCIS with large clear margins; others do not. Some surgeons insist on MRI of the breast after core needle biopsy; others do not. Some surgeons insist on lymph node biopsy; others do not. Some surgeons insist on breast irradiation; others do not. Regarding the biology of breast cancer described before, side effects and harms of standard treatment of DCIS leads us to the following:

Harmless Alternative Treatment of DCIS

1. DCIS is detected by screening mammography and diagnosed by pathologist on core needle biopsy of the lesion. The patient should have MRI of the breast and genetic test of the lesion.
2. MRI of the breast is indispensable because (a) it determines the resectability of the lesion and its extension, (b) it rules out other associated foci multicentricity or multilocality, (c) it avoids misclassification of DCIS versus invasive, (d) one-time MRI will serve also as a baseline image, which is very important in future follow-ups, and (e) if MRI does not show any invasive foci, no more biopsy, no lymph node sampling.
3. Oncotype Dx, RS less than 55 (low risk, encompassing majority of DCIS).
4. Definitive surgery, hook wire localization of the lesion. Large number of local recurrence is due to incomplete excision of DCIS. In order to alleviate that, two to four hook wires (as we described before) should be inserted into the breast, targeting and bracketing microcalcifications or the marker deployed at the site of biopsy during the core needle biopsy. The entire lesion should be removed at least with 1 cm clear margin at the first surgical attempt proven by x-ray specimen and pathology. This prevents largely local breast cancer recurrence.
5. No lymph node biopsy, no breast irradiation.

Comments: We have seen in one case without MRI at first surgical attempt that clear margin could not be obtained. In the second attempt, however, clear margin was reported by the pathologist. The patient, frustrated by two surgeries, requested mastectomy. Mastectomy showed residual, not only at the vicinity of the DCIS but also microscopic foci at some distances. With correct bracketing technique and MRI, surgeons often can get the whole cancer out. A successful surgery oncologically and cosmetically depends on the skill and experience of the radiologist and the surgeon. Once DCIS is treated surgically with 1 cm clear margins, no radiation is indicated because of the following:

1. No impact on survival.
2. Difficulty of diagnosis of local recurrence, very important.
3. Numerous minor and major side effects reported previously in irradiated breast.
4. In case of local recurrence, patient loses her breast (mastectomy).

STANDARD TREATMENT OF INVASIVE BREAST CANCER: MASTECTOMY

"Mastectomy is indicated in any type of invasive breast cancer." However, it was found that mastectomy is unnecessary in large numbers of invasive breast cancer. The majority of surgeons are in agreement in two issues:

First, mastectomy is indicated in nonresectable breast cancer (advanced or inflammatory invasive breast cancer).

Second, simple mastectomy is indicated instead of radical or super-radical mastectomy.

STANDARD OF CONSERVATIVE TREATMENT OF INVASIVE BREAST CANCER

This standard is based on TNM classifications. "It consists of lumpectomy, axillary lymph node biopsy, if it is metastatic, axillary lymph node dissection and followed by chemotherapy and breast irradiation." In previous chapters we saw that variant of surgical treatment of the breast, lymph node dissection, and breast irradiation had no impact on survival but caused serious side effects and irreparable damages and harm to the patient. This led us to the following:

Alternative Harmless Treatment of Invasive Breast Cancer

This treatment is based on genetic findings of breast cancer.

1. When suspicious lesions are found by imaging techniques or by palpation and diagnosed as cancer by pathologist on core needle biopsy, patient should have genetic test of mammaprint of cancer and breast MRI, which can show the extension of the lesion and its resectability and presence or absence of other foci of lesion.
2. In case of monofocal cancer, two to four hook wires should be used for localization of the lesion, taking into account its extension on MRI surgical removal with at least 1 cm clear margin at first surgical attempt.
3. If genetic test of cancerous lesion shows that cancer is high risk for metastasis it indicates first, body MRI, if positive, PET scan of the whole body, then chemotherapy. Therefore, no axillary lymph node sampling. Genetic test surrogates lymph node sampling and lymph node dissection. If genetic test shows cancer is in low risk for distant metastasis regardless of the size of cancer, no further treatment is necessary than its removal. Eventually, anti-hormone therapy, if the lesion is hormone receptor positive and the patient can tolerate the side effects.

As we can see, three classical procedures—lymph node sampling, lymph node dissection, and breast radiation—are omitted because of the serious side effects and complications. Particularly, breast irradiation by destruction of breast tissue causes deformity and fibrosis, which prevents detection of local recurrences.

Comparison of classic standard conservative treatment versus alternative harmless treatment

First Example: Patient, forty-eight years old, on her left screening mammography, a small 8 mm lesion was found and proved to be invasive. Patient underwent lumpectomy and breast irradiation. Six years later, clinically a mass was found at the site of previous surgery, but mammography showed no distinct lesion. Biopsy showed 3 cm invasive cancer, three and a half times bigger than the original breast cancer treated with mastectomy.

At least 30% of breast cancer recurrence is detected by palpable mass, not by mammography.

Despite that, the proponents of breast irradiation consider it as prophylactic tool, then the question arises, why not irradiate the opposite breast, which is in high risk (68%) for developing breast cancer?

Before radiation   After radiation

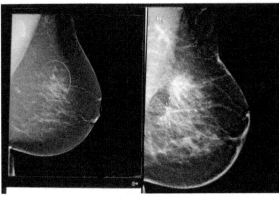

Figure 16.2. Mammography shows after radiation skin thickening, intense fibrotic scar, shadowing the entire structure of the breast. How is it possible to detect breast cancer recurrence?

16.1   16.2

Figure 16.1. Left screening mammography showed small mass density (in the circle); biopsy invasive breast cancer, patient had lumpectomy and radiation. Follow-up mammography (fig. 16.2) showed dense breast; no new lesion can be detected.

For the physician who believes that recurrence can be a new source of metastasis, they should know that the radiation of the breast impede early detection of recurrence.

Second Example: In 1984, patient at the age of forty-seven had a 2 cm well-differentiated (good prognosis) invasive left breast cancer. Patient had lumpectomy and breast radiation. Patient was followed up annually. Patient at the age of seventy-two, twenty-seven years after treatment, because of focal tissue distortion on her left mammography, MRI of the breast was requested, which demonstrated small mass far from the mammographic changes. The biopsy revealed invasive breast cancer; mastectomy showed 4 mm well-differentiated invasive breast cancer. Patient at the age of seventy-two lost her breast because of fortuitous MRI finding. However, this small lesion could be removed, avoiding mastectomy and its indelible scar. But that procedure is considered unorthodox treatment, violating the standard of care (fig. 16.3).

Mammography MRI

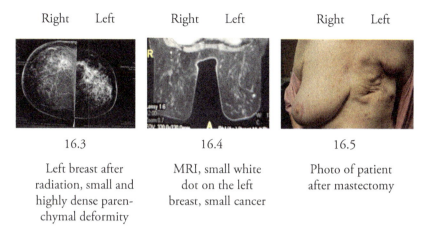

16.3	16.4	16.5
Left breast after radiation, small and highly dense parenchymal deformity	MRI, small white dot on the left breast, small cancer	Photo of patient after mastectomy

It should be noted that when surgical removal of recurrence in irradiated breast is attempted, it is not without healing problems; irradiated breast is virtually half dead.

First example of harmless conservative treatment without radiation of invasive breast cancer:

In September 2002 screening mammography showed small mass density of 8 mm in the outer upper quadrant of the left breast; lesion removed by hook wire localization showed well-differentiated invasive breast cancer, no radiation of the breast (fig. 16.6).

In October 2003 follow-up mammography showed scar density at the site of the previous surgery (fig. 16.7).

In June 2006 follow-up mammography showed disappearance of the scar and appearance of small mass (fig. 16.8). Surgery showed recurrent 4 mm cancer much smaller than the original cancer. If the patient had radiation, this recurrence could not have been detected so small on mammography, with such a good cosmetics results of the breast (fig. 16.9). This patient preserved her breast and again no breast irradiation. The last time this patient was seen six years after radiation, no sign of recurrence was seen in follow-up on either side.

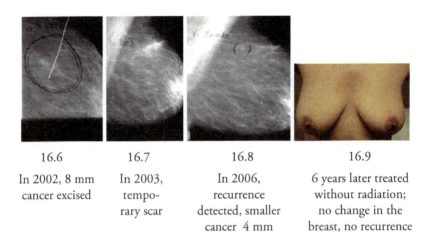

16.6	16.7	16.8	16.9
In 2002, 8 mm cancer excised	In 2003, temporary scar	In 2006, recurrence detected, smaller cancer 4 mm	6 years later treated without radiation; no change in the breast, no recurrence

Second Example:

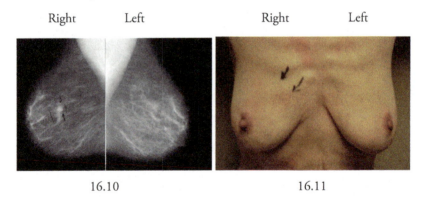

16.10	16.11
Patient, 62-year-old, small white nodule (small arrows on the right side) proved to be a small invasive cancer; patient had total excision of the lesion and no radiation.	Photography, 8 years later, good cosmetic results arrows at the site of excision; no sign of recurrence

COMPARISON OF ALTERNATIVE TREATMENT OF BREAST CANCER

Classic treatment	Alternative treatment
BASED ON CLASSICAL TNM	BASED ON GENETIC TEST
Classic paradigms	Genetic paradigms
No genetic test of cancer	Core needle biopsy genetic test of cancer
Total resection of cancer	Total resection of cancer
Axillary sentinel lymph node sampling (surgery)	No lymph node sampling (no surgery)
Axillary lymph node dissection (surgery)	No axillary lymph node dissection (no surgery)
Complications of lymph node dissection	No complications of lymph node dissection
Chemotherapy if lymph node metastasis	No chemotherapy if cancer low risk
Chemotherapy if size of cancer > 1 cm	Chemotherapy if cancer is high risk
Breast irradiation	No breast irradiation
Complications and side effects of radiation	No complication
Follow-up for detection of recurrence, tedious and very expensive	Follow-up simple, not expensive
Delay in the detection of recurrence, if detected, bigger than the original cancer	No delay, recurrence detected smaller than original cancer
Cosmetically, long term mediocre to poor	Cosmetically excellent, normal
Patient satisfaction low or average	Patient satisfaction good to excellent
Cost of treatment and follow-up very high	Cost of treatment and follow-up very low

| Survival the same | Survival the same |
| Breast reconstruction difficult or not feasible | Breast reconstruction easy, always feasible |

Summary of the following acts should be performed for harmless conservative treatment of breast cancer.

1. Diagnosis of breast cancer should be confirmed on core needle biopsy.
2. After core needle biopsy, all patients should have genetic test of cancer if pathologic diagnosis is intraductal carcinoma, oncotype Dx, and if diagnosis is invasive breast cancer mammaprint (symphony) should be requested.
3. Patient should have a contrasted MRI of the breasts, which determines the resectability of cancer and rules out the presence of other foci. For invasive breast cancer with high risk for metastasis, request whole body MRI. If breast cancer is monofocal, proceed to localization for surgery.
4. Nonpalpable breast cancer is localized by two to four hook wire by the radiologist for the surgeon.
5. The surgeon is guided by the hook wire and should remove the entire lesion with at least 1 cm clear margin at the first surgical attempt, then proceed to plastic remodeling if necessary.
6. In DCIS and in invasive cancer, no sentinel lymph node sampling, no lymph node dissection, no radiation. In genetically low risk for distant metastasis, no chemotherapy. In high-risk systemic, chemotherapy is indicated.
7. In case of local recurrence, the same above algorithm should be repeated. If the lesion is resectable, it will be removed and the breast preserved. If the lesion is extensive, nonresectable, mastectomy and reconstruction is easily feasible. For recurrences, surgery can be repeated like surgery in multiple bilateral fibroadenomas.

CHAPTER 17

FOLLOW-UP PROGRAM OF PATIENT TREATED FOR BREAST CANCER WHO HAS NO SYMPTOMS

Today, there is no rational standard for follow-up for patients treated for breast cancer. The present program of follow-up is an arbitrary regimen practiced mainly after conservative treatment (lumpectomy plus radiation). Some surgeons schedule to see the patient every six months, radiotherapist every four months, oncologist every four months, radiologist every six months for five years.

Why this rush? The argument is to detect the recurrence of breast cancer as soon as possible. In the matter of breast cancer, there is no race against time. Clinical and biological data show that the majority of breast cancer developing silently and evolving for years from molecular to microscopic, then from microscopic to clinical radiological detectable lesion; all these years we were not concerned about breast cancer. Now, suddenly months of delay to detect the recurrence becomes a matter of concern. It should be said that clinical trials and genetic findings show detection of local recurrence of invasive breast cancer sooner or later has no impact on survival; the outcome of patient is determined before the detection of primary breast cancer. On the other hand, as far as clinical follow-up for distant metastasis is concerned, it is also reported in the literature: patients treated for breast cancer were divided in two groups. One group was followed up by oncologic program—tight visits, particularly using expensive tools such as blood test, chest x-ray, bone scan for detection of distant breast cancer recurrence. The result and survival were no different than the group of patients who were seen by general practitioners without oncologic regimen. This trial is very important; it shows that even when occult distant metastasis (early detection of metastasis) in asymptomatic patients (patients without signs of disease) is discovered, it has no impact on survival when compared with the other group who did not have oncological follow-up. However, the interval visits by oncologist is justified when patients have chemotherapy in order to treat its side effects and check for metastasis.

Follow-up of treated breast cancer treated by harmless alternative method based on genetics screening breast cancer

It is simple, precise, and inexpensive.

Patient had MRI in the beginning of the treatment, which allowed alternative methods. If original DCIS or invasive breast cancer were in low risk for recurrence, patient can have annual physical examination and screening mammography.

If DCIS and invasive breast cancer were in high risk, patient can have annual oncologic consultation (physical examination, screening mammography, eventually blood test for biomarker, MRI, PET/CT scan). Oncologic workup can be instituted only if any suspicious sign develops after primary treatment.

Treatment of local recurrence

In our conservative alternative treatment, in case of local recurrence, the same procedure will be used as for the primary. After any local breast cancer recurrence, genetic test of the lesion should be done. It may change the nature of the treatment. For example, if the patient has been treated for the primary invasive cancer with Tamoxifen, the recurrence may turn to hormone receptor negative. At this time, the patient can be treated with chemotherapy and no more by anti-hormone therapy, or if original cancer DCIS or invasive breast cancer was in low risk and recurrent as low risk, again proceed to total re-excision. If original cancer DCIS or invasive cancer was in low risk for recurrence and now the recurrent cancer is of high risk, chemotherapy is indicated; still the patient can preserve her breast.

In summary, in terms of local breast cancer recurrence, as long as it is resectable and does not affect inacceptable cosmesis of the breast, excision and re-excision for recurrence can be repeated, and if it is not resectable, mastectomy and reconstruction are easily feasible contrary to irradiated breast. Remember that survival is not affected by variety of local treatment in invasive breast cancer nor by its local recurrence. It is affected by other factors, mainly genetic signature of the primary breast cancer and genetic signature of the local breast cancer recurrence.

Compromised guideline would be the following for breast cancer screening:

1. Patients at the age of thirty to forty with BRC1, BRC2 positive (with 80% lifetime risk), annual physical examination, MRI every two years (invasive cancer is common in BRC positive, MRI detects it sooner than mammography), and after the age of forty, if no prophylactic procedure is done, add annual screening mammography. Mammography is gold for detection of DCIS. MRI is platinum for detection of invasive breast cancer.
2. Patients after the age of forty with family history (25% risk of breast cancer) with dense breasts, lumpy tissue with advanced fibrocystic condition, numerous cyst aspirations, and multiple biopsies, annual physical examination, screening mammography, and MRI every two years.
3. General population, 13% lifetime risk of cancer after the age of forty, annual physical examination and annual screening mammography. In dense breasts add ultrasonography and MRI at the discretion of the physicians.
4. After conservative treatment of breast cancer, if lesion was in low risk, annual physical examination and mammography; if in high risk, annual of oncological workup.

Thus a large number of breast cancer will not be missed. First beneficiary would be the patient and second the radiologist because of the decrease of the risk of liability.

CHAPTER 18

FINAL NOTES

SURVIVAL OF BREAST CANCER

One of the most historical demonstrations of breast cancer outcome was the work of J. Dawson et al. published from the University of Chicago Hospital in the *Journal of Cancer* in 1982, on their experience on 746 patients treated with mastectomy between 1929 and 1955. Of these patients 107 survived twenty-five years, and they compared these patients with the control group who died in a median three to four years after diagnosis of cancer. They found the following:

1. Majority of twenty-five-year survival were younger at the time of diagnosis, less than fifty years old with a cancer smaller than 2 cm with more grade 1 tumor with less lymphatic involvement.
2. Most important and amazing finding, 12% of twenty-five-year survival had original tumor more than 5 cm. 11% of patients had four or more lymph node metastasis at the original treatment, and 63% of the patient had lymphatic and vascular invasion within the tumor or lymph node involvement at the original surgery.

The authors concluded that they were not able to accurately predict who would be expected to survive twenty-five years or who would die within four years. This was their statement thirty-three years ago and is still the same today.

We learn from this remarkable work:

1. Breast cancer patients treated by surgery alone (mastectomy) can survive twenty-five years after the worst type of breast cancer without radiation and without chemotherapy.
2. No patient should be desperate because their cancer is in advanced stage. They may live another twenty-five years or more, particularly with much more efficient systemic therapy that we have today in our arsenal and much more coming in the future.

ANSWERS TO THE QUESTIONS

In the term of this book, we have to answer questions that we have posed at the beginning of this book. Can we prevent breast cancer?

As a general rule, as long as we don't know the cause of the disease, we cannot prevent it. Breast cancer is not an exception. However, in medicine, there are many diseases with unknown cause that have been treated and have been prevented or reduced the risk of occurrence of the diseases.

1. In hereditary breast cancer, due to damage of BRC1/BRC2 genes, we cannot prevent the transmission of the genes from parents to the offspring unless we examine the eggs formed by parents in the laboratory and examine them genetically, discarding the eggs with the damaged genes and inseminating the healthy egg to the mother or to a surrogate mother. Otherwise, once the damaged genes are transmitted to the offspring, then we can only reduce the risk of occurrence of breast cancer from 85% to 5%, ovarian cancer from 40% to 5% by bilateral mastectomy and bilateral oophorectomy.
2. Breast cancer caused by ethnical factors: Risk of breast cancer is higher in some ethnicities such as in Jewish

Ashkenazim, Eskimos; no prevention in the horizon, but intermarriage between different ethnic groups may reduce the risk of breast cancer.
3. Reducing breast cancer risk by environmental factors: The best known is exposure to x-ray before the age of thirty. Therefore, exposure to x-ray and radioactive material and carcinogenic substance should be avoided as much as possible.
4. Risk reduction by medication: Medications tooted as preventative of breast cancer experimented were Avista and Tamoxifen. Preventing obesity, avoiding tobacco and alcohol, using healthy foods, and regular exercise provide us the same amount of risk reduction as so-called preventive medications.

CAN WE CURE BREAST CANCER?

WHAT IS THE DEFINITION OF THE CURE IN BREAST CANCER?

1. Statistical cure

2. Clinical cure

If a woman of fifty years is treated for breast cancer and we get total disappearance of symptoms of the disease, including metastasis, then living and dying like her normal healthy sibling, this is statistical cure.

What is clinical cure? Total disappearance of symptoms of the disease after treatment for a period of time, months or decades, but finally cancer recurs. Patient may succumb to breast cancer metastasis or other diseases.

As we said previously, for breast cancer prevention, treatment and cure of the disease become possible when the cause is known. In the last century, the causes of a large number of diseases discovered either were viral, bacterial, fungal, or parasitic; their prevention and cure were obtained by vaccines or anti-viral, anti-fungal, anti-bacterial, anti-parasitic, anti-septic drugs. All epithelial breast cancer began from inside of the milk ducts, ductal carcinoma in situ (DCIS) progenitor of invasive breast cancer. Despite unknown cause, by its total eradication, not only can we cure DCIS, but also we might prevent to a large extent the development and appearance of invasive breast cancer, thus reducing mortality.

What about invasive breast cancer?

In 1972, Mustagalio from Finland published his thirty-year experience on 709 invasive breast cancer patients treated by lumpectomy and radiation and concluded that breast cancer is a general systemic disease from onset and is incurable.

In 1990, Haybittle reported the only way to assess cure of breast cancer is to show that the risk of dying or force of mortality after treatment parallels the expected mortality of normal population and called it statistical cure. No controlled trial had yet reported providing cure for invasive breast cancer. That was the conclusion in the last century, but the trend is different in the twenty-first century. Because of progress in medicine, and particularly in the science of genetics, today we are able to foresee the occurrence of breast cancer in patients with family history. By genetic test we can discover damage of BRC1/BRC2 genes. We also treat a large number of diseases without knowing their causes. We can also cure diseases with known cause without targeting or treating the cause. Each year, half a million of people die of heart attacks in the USA because of vascular lesions. It does not mean that everyone with a heart attack will die. Today, a large number of patients with massive heart attack get angioplasty or stent, and the signs and discomfort disappear despite the fact that one-third of their heart is damaged and nonfunctional. However, <u>we get clinical cure, which may last decades,</u> without the underlying cause of the heart attack being treated (vascular disease). In breast cancer, the situation is still better despite the fact that we do not know the cause. A genetic test can show us that either cancer is in low risk or high risk for metastasis. Low risk for metastasis in invasive breast cancer is luminal A. By removing the entire cancer tissue, 90% of the patients are clinically cured. Genetic test can warn us of the risk of distant metastasis, not detectable by our most sophisticated tools, but if present microscopically, they are more vulnerable to chemotherapy than when detectable (overt metastasis). We may obtain most likely much longer clinical cure when metastasis is treated in occult stage.

Genetics can determine what the driver of cancer machinery is. If we cannot destroy the engine of cancer, we can target and paralyze the driver and gain again long clinical cure.

In conclusion, today, because of genetic revolution, we can cure clinically a large number of breast cancer without any harm.

Harm from surgery can easily be avoided—correct lumpectomy, no axillary lymph node sampling, no dissection.

Harm from radiation can easily be eliminated—no radiation in conservative treatment.

Harm from anti-hormone therapy can easily be prevented, if not tolerated.

Harm from chemotherapy can be avoidable if genetic test is performed; in low risk, 60% of patients can be dispensed of chemotherapy.

Last question: Why is the treatment of breast cancer so expensive?

In the mass media as well as in many medical publications, high cost of breast cancer treatment is attributed to overdiagnosis and overtreatment. Overdiagnosis means detection of a large number of benign lesions or slow-growing breast cancer by imaging technique mammography and MRI for which patients undergo harsh, expensive, unnecessary treatment. In previous chapters we saw the benefit of overdiagnosis by MRI. In fact, that is not overdiagnosis that increases the cost; that is overtreatment, because all breast cancers are treated the same way (one size fits all). Treatment of breast cancer is not yet based on modern genetic findings. The following are the reasons why physicians do not apply genetic tests in the treatment of breast cancer:

1. Unaware of the benefits of genetic tests
2. Aware of genetic test but uncertain of the results
3. Treatment of breast cancer upon the genetic tests not being publicized as standard, therefore not practiced generally because of apprehension of liability

In the last decades we learn from numerous randomized clinical trials that many procedures used in the treatment of breast cancer are unnecessary, which still are performed. With that in mind, genetic discovery compels us to adopt a new policy in the treatment of breast cancer (alternative treatment).

How can we reduce the enormous cost of breast cancer treatment?

If breast cancer was detected more in situ stage or smaller invasive breast cancer.

If breast cancer was diagnosed by core needle biopsy.

If patient had MRI of the breast and genetic test of cancer after core needle biopsy.

If radiologist had localized cancer by two to four hook wires.

If surgeon could remove the entire breast cancer at first surgical attempt with clear margins.

If oncologist had based chemotherapy on genetic test, in 40% to 60% of breast cancer regardless of the size and status of the lymph node, patients could be spared from chemotherapy.

If axillary lymph node sampling and axillary lymph node dissection were restricted and surrogated by genetic test, complications and arm lymphedema could be prevented.

If irradiation of the breast cancer that has no impact on survival could be eliminated.

If oncologic follow-up was based on genetic test, unnecessary PET/CT scan could be avoided.

If unnecessary tight follow-up visits of patients without complaints every six months for five years were restricted to annual visits.

All this will contribute to huge cost reduction (in order of billion dollars for society) in the treatment of breast cancer and more well-being of patients.

At the close of this book, remembering the prophetic statement of some physicians in the past, Hyes Agnew in the eighteenth century said, "I don't despair of carcinoma being cured somewhat in the future but this blessed achievement will never be wrought of the knife of the surgeon." Dr. George Crile (1970), forty-five years ago, wrote, "Women should know about treatment of breast cancer that mastectomy, axillary lymph node dissection and breast irradiation are unnecessary." All proven to be true today.

CPSIA information can be obtained
at www.ICGtesting.com
Printed in the USA
LVOW05s1917300416
486091LV00045B/943/P